# TWO TURNS FROM ZERO

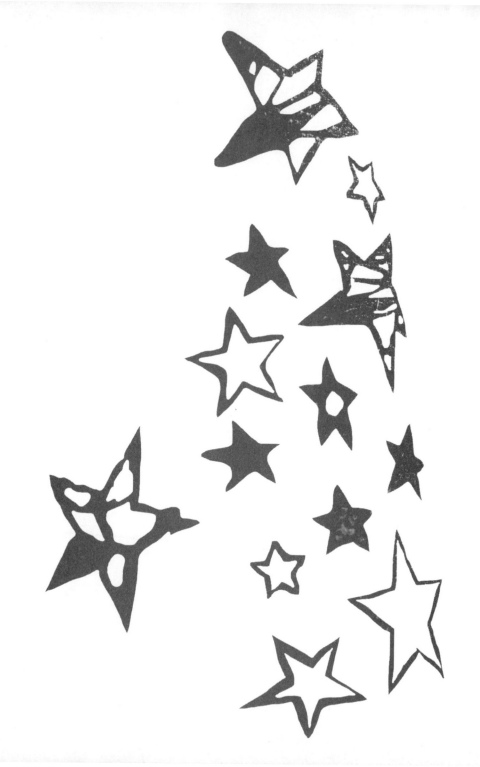

# TWO TURNS FROM ZERO

## PUSHING TO HIGHER FITNESS GOALS—CONVERTING THEM TO LIFE STRENGTH

## STACEY GRIFFITH

WITH KAREN MOLINE

*wm*

WILLIAM MORROW
*An Imprint of HarperCollinsPublishers*

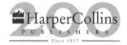

This book is written as a source of information only. The information contained in this book should by no means be considered a substitute for the advice of a qualified medical professional, who should always be consulted before beginning any new diet, exercise, or other health program.

All efforts have been made to ensure the accuracy of the information contained in this book as of the date published. The author and the publisher expressly disclaim responsibility for any adverse effects arising from the use or application of the information contained herein or for any injuries suffered or damages or losses incurred as a result of following the exercise program in this book.

All photographs are from the author's personal collection except for pages 61, 138, 169, 222, 231, 266, 333: Debby Hymowitz; page 3: Erin Howitt; page 13: Jill Lotenberg; page 175: Robert Pargac; page 194: Chris Fanning; and page 355: Sean Simes.

HarperCollins books may be purchased for educational, business, or sales promotional use. For information please e-mail the Special Markets Department at SPsales@harpercollins.com.

A hardcover edition of this book was published in 2017 by William Morrow, an imprint of HarperCollins Publishers.

FIRST WILLIAM MORROW PAPERBACK EDITION PUBLISHED 2017.

Designed by Bonni Leon-Berman

Library of Congress Cataloging-in-Publication Data has been applied for.

ISBN 978-0-06-249685-0

17 18 19 20 21  LSC  10 9 8 7 6 5 4 3 2 1

*I dedicate this book to my junior high school "Boys Sports"*
*PE teacher, Mr. Bob Hunter.*

His countless classes taught me that my body would be the greatest tool I would ever own, that physically "learning" how to fall was a thing, that quitting was not an option, that I could still play even if I didn't feel great, that exercise was medicine, and that being the only girl in a boys-only class meant I could believe I was destined for greatness.

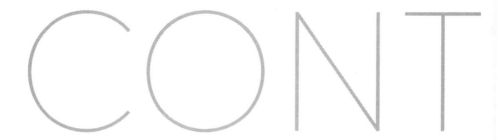

# CONT

# ENTS

# AUTHOR'S NOTE

I could not have written this book without the help of Karen Moline. She helped me organize my "Post-it note" thoughts and showed me what parts of my own story would be interesting and would fit within the message I wanted to send about fitness and motivation. Her insights are found on every page of this book, and I can't thank her enough.

"You can't get what you want by always taking the easy path."

# INTRODUCTION
# FIND YOUR
# ULTIMATE
# CENTER

Imagine you have the control and motivation to change the direction of your life . . . today, *now,* in this moment.

Imagine that today you cross over into a new level of creative thinking that sends you marching toward outrageous personal success.

Imagine you'll finally live the dream you always wished could come true. Imagine yourself *finally* embracing a physical method, combined with some amazing visualization techniques, that increases your self-motivation and provides you with a greater sense of inner calm, spirit, joy, and love.

Would you be willing to take a look?

That's what you will find in *Two Turns from Zero*. This is not only what I tell my students at SoulCycle—to crank up that resistance knob to a place where they can push past their personal best. It's also what you turn when you go from zero—a blank page full of possibilities—into a whole new world of physical and creative self-discovery.

The first turn is to deal with the stuff going on in your head (the what, why, and when you want to change your life—we'll get to that later in the book).

The second turn gets at how you're going to take the good ideas you have about yourself and your future and turn them into the kind of *action* that will always get the results you want and need.

And the whole thing together—*Two Turns from Zero*—is my life mantra:

You can't get what you want by always taking the easiest path. So turn it up Two from Zero, and let's go . . . Are you ready? *Come on!*

I am a Senior Master Instructor at SoulCycle in New York City, and I've taught to sold-out classes all over the country. My students have joked that it was easier getting into Studio 54 in its heyday than it is to get into my classes. These classes have become so popular because my students know they're going to get my unique mix of a hard-core workout for their bodies and my even harder workout for their hearts, minds, and spirit. I don't mess around, and not a minute is wasted. And they know it.

I've been at this for more than two decades, so I've mastered my coaching style. I'm flattered when people say I'm the Tony Robbins of exercise: a combination of the mindful focus of Deepak Chopra, the exuberant high energy of Kelly Ripa, and the cool sexiness of Pink. When I teach from the floor, I

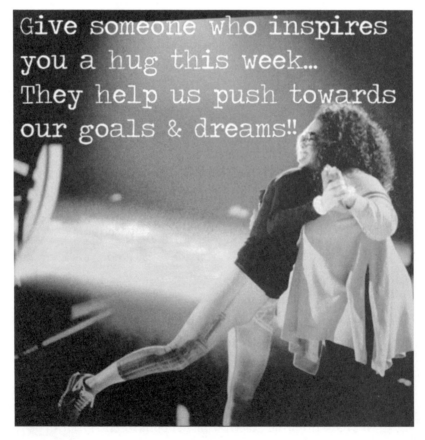

Me and O

become a combination of comedienne, spiritual guide, motivator, and "entertrainer" (a phrase I coined when asked to describe myself!).

Those comparisons make me blush! But I *do* know I know how to motivate my students. It all comes together through my highly charged blend of music, positive mantras, and intense exercise sequences. I expect their butts to be up off those bike seats. That's what gets their abs taut, their triceps firm, and their hearts pumping—and it's what triggers that deliriously wonderful explosion of endorphins.

Most of all, I know my students are there to give it their all—and they want the same from me. They expect results. They *demand* results. So do I.

I wish I could say I was born knowing this, but I learned what works the hard way. The *very* hard way. Looking at me now, it's hard to believe I was once a drug addict, an alcoholic, a smoker, a liar, and a very sad and messed-up person. But I was.

What saved me? *Exercise.* It made me accountable to myself by teaching me how to feel strong. But I don't mean just on the outside. It got to me in a deeper way by showing me how to have a healthy relationship with myself. The strength of my muscles empowered the strength of my feelings, thoughts, hopes, and expectations. And exercise also became a time when I nourished myself by being with other people who had the same goals.

It's hard to define exactly what happens when a group of people get together and *move,* but there's a shared momentum and motivation that drive everyone forward, and everyone feels bonded in the process. I found it invigorating, and it helped me run toward the life I craved and to stop making excuses.

I will say more about this later, but over time, exercise helped me turn my life around. And believe me . . . you can, too.

In my life today, I lead a posse of students who are dripping with sweat and filled with adrenaline after each class. And as a result, they are happier, more relaxed human beings than they ever have been before. Yes, they are physically stronger because I push them to get results they never thought they would achieve. But while they were on that journey to getting there, I helped them see an emotional strength in themselves that they didn't know was possible. What they discover is a side of themselves they never knew.

By getting in the best shape of their lives, they merge the joy of physical movement with personal goals and fulfillment. They discover that they possess a potent power to speeding up their journey toward their goals and dreams.

*Two Turns from Zero* is here to teach you how to harness that power, at home, in your own time. This book is your private coach, and with it in your hands, you will embark on your own personal journey of transformation. You can do this on your own. No bike necessary! No gym needed! Or you can do what I did and find your squad while you pull it together at home!

To help you on your way to mastery, I have an approach I call LET. It stands for Love, Eat, Train. And just like the shampoo instructions, I add in the word *Repeat* because you've got to do it over and over again if you want it to work. If you follow LET—with lots of repeats—you find what I call your Ultimate Center. We all strive to live inside this centered place—where we are strong and laser-focused. In this Ultimate Center, we achieve the balance of core emotional strength we all need to face whatever crap life throws our way. Being there keeps us stable, sturdy, happy, healthy, and fulfilled, even in the face of unexpected heartache or problems.

A lot of exercise teachers and coaches tell their students that the way to feel better about themselves is to change their outside appearance. I don't buy that approach. It's never worked for me, so I don't see how it can work for others. I believe exactly the opposite—true change comes from the inside out. Sure, we all feel better about ourselves if we're happy with the way we look. But people don't really change the way they look until they feel different deep inside.

Only then can you achieve lasting results that will take you to that Ultimate Center. And now we're back to taking two turns from zero. As you'll see in this book, it takes more than just a resistance knob you turn on an indoor cycling bike to make you push harder.

*Two Turns from Zero* is about discovering that working out isn't just the key to athleticism or stronger muscles. It's about having a new relationship with *yourself*. The kind of relationship you enjoy being in.

I'm also going to introduce you to one of my favorite sayings. It's something I call AOA—Adult-Onset Athleticism. I love it because it means you can become an athlete at any age, and being an athlete doesn't mean you have to be involved in team sports. (More on this when I get into training later in the book.)

I've written this book because so many people are filled with a desire for change, but they can't stick to the action plan that will bring them long-lasting results. I have been starting my classes with "Two turns from zero" since I began teaching indoor cycling in 1996. It stuck, and it resonates. It's a metaphor for my life. I want you to use it to help you discover what *you* need. I want you to figure out what movement turns you on so you'll stick to it. When you find it, it will keep you motivated for life.

By the time you finish reading this book, you'll be using my coaching strategies to figure out who's really calling the shots in your life. I'll ruin the suspense: It will be you! (Don't worry—you won't be alone. We'll get to your all-important squad!)

Following the steps I've laid out in this book will give you the confidence to say, proudly, that *you're* the one to get your life flowing. You are the one who gets you through every challenge you face. It's about believing in all your talents and abilities. It's about becoming emotionally strong and resilient—*that* is what allows you to get into the best shape of your life.

All you need is the right coach. I'm here jumping off the pages with my fist in the air, cheering you on—with fresh ideas and methods that work. Let me *entertrain* you!

I've taught thousands of students since I started my coaching career, which began in earnest when I fell in love with the indoor cycling bike and became an instructor in 1996. Then, in 2006, I met Julie Rice and Elizabeth Cutler, and they told me they wanted to create a yoga-based spiritual journey on the bike—what became SoulCycle—and we just clicked. They saw how I taught—a unique method based on my instincts, my previous teaching experience as a fitness instructor, and my cardio-party attitude. We gave riders the freedom to dance on the bike. Our movement, passion, and formula had never been used before, and SoulCycle quickly expanded from one ground-floor-lobby studio that had a rickshaw in the front so people could find it to the most popular indoor cycling chain in the world, with thirty studios in New York City, almost twenty in Los Angeles, and many more to come.

When the SoulCycle craze hit, everyone tried to understand its secret sauce. Why were hardworking New Yorkers hovering over their computers every Monday at noon, vying to secure a bike in a class with their favorite instructor? It was due to the entire experience they had in our classes. It wasn't just a hardcore workout for their muscles. Riders left feeling uplifted and *transformed* in every possible way.

They may have come to class wanting a firmer butt—and they got it!—but they soon learned that firmer resolutions needed to change as well. Students come to class with all the challenges and stresses of their lives. Some are in mourning, or they are coming from a chemo treatment. Others are in the ecstasies of love! I also have students who come to me determined to finally lose those pounds they've struggled with all their lives. Or some just want to shed the baby weight or look buff for a special event. I see my students pedaling hard and feeling the joy that comes from exerting their bodies and pushing themselves further. But most important, they tell me how they are able to translate this feeling into making real changes in dealing with their lives.

I push them because they come in wanting to be pushed. They make me so proud, because they prove that easy doesn't change you. You change through determination and hard work.

If you take the time to think about the difficult decisions you've made in your life, you will realize how much stronger you were after making them. Now you can look back at what you endured and tell yourself, "Wow, I can't believe I got through that. Look where I am now!"

I also learned that to be the most effective teacher possible I had to get off the podium bike. I walk around the room now, keeping my eye on everyone. This way, I feel the vibe. I can correct someone who may be having an off day, or I can help someone reach higher. With this laser focus on teaching and coaching, I can be the "Entertrainer." All my teaching comes from love, empowerment, and laughter, helping my students learn how to enjoy the power of movement while keeping mental negativity from getting in the way.

I want my students to come right up against themselves, to pedal hard to the top of the mountain . . . past fears, insecurities, bad habits, procrastination, self-criticism, and inde-cision . . . to come down the other side into the clear stretch of accomplished joy. "Two turns from zero" is a metaphor for beating the challenges we are trying to push past. It's facing and overcoming the issues in our tissues—the deep-seated memories and learned behavior we get hung up on.

We all have those awful nagging voices in our heads that say we're no good or we can't do it or we'll never make it. I'm here to help you with those nagging voices, and we'll discuss that throughout this book. It's a really important issue, because no matter what, you can never give up. We will set goals, and we will hit them. That's the moment we turn into the goal, and we hit *that*. We never stop scoring goals for the rest of our lives together. As coach and athlete, let's kick ass together. Cool?

That's why this book is about *change*—which happens when you build mental and physical muscles. It's also about finding the magic connection between intention and action. About training your emotions and your purpose. About clearing out the mental negativity and getting out of your own way. I have called on my own painful journey of personal transformation to create a unique method for personal empowerment, com-bining newfound physical strength, mental resolve, and joy-ful intention.

This method will teach you how to channel your *inner ath-lete* as I've learned to channel mine. I want you to embrace and love the body you were born into as I have learned to love mine, even though I abused it with my addictions. I want to help you find your purpose, then embrace it so you can follow your self-proclaimed path in the most inspirational and joyful manner possible. I want you to have all the love you deserve and to give back the love you feel in return.

This book contains the tools for finding your true, authentic power, for keeping your body and mind in motion, for always moving forward, and for taking on life as you have never taken it on before.

One of my favorite sayings is "You are stronger than you were yesterday, but no way are you as strong as you'll be tomorrow." Another one is "Now, let's crush it." So, let's crush it!

## HOW TO USE THIS BOOK

I always say Motivation = Intention + Action. This book shows you how to get motivation by finding your purpose, and then set your intentions for change before committing to my action plan.

The first chapter in part I tells you about the ups and downs of my life, so you'll see what I did wrong and how I learned to make it right—turning my flaws, addictions, and shame into strength and balance. Along the way, I was able to train my heart to open up to the love I knew I deserved. I also found my true purpose in life, which gave me the motivation to change. I will discuss why everyone needs a purpose in life, and how, when you live with purpose, you can commit to making healthy changes.

Whatever it is that is holding you back, once you read my story I hope you will be inspired and know you can do it, too. In part II, I will show you how to set your intentions, as well as the basics of defining goals, which everyone must master before tackling the journey to finding their Ultimate Center. I'll also introduce you to Moving Meditation and show you how it works. Next I will describe creative visualizations to help you focus and move forward. Read the Moving Meditations and creative visualizations all the way through before doing them. From there I will help you clear the physical and mental clutter so you can make a fresh start.

In part III, I will show you my LET program: Love, Eat, Train. Living from your Ultimate Center can only happen when you learn to love yourself and realize you deserve to be loved. There's a really important chapter next. It's called Eat, and it's important because we all do it. I use this chapter to tell you about my unique approach to food. You are going to replace your old eating habits with good new ones, and when you do, you're going to reach that goal weight. I will address nutrition basics with menu lists and some of my favorite recipes, all with a Stacey G twist.

I know you've been waiting for this next chapter. It's called Train, and it's one of my favorite topics. I'm going to lay out what you need to know about the benefits of exercise (and good sleep) and then show you how to train your body the Stacey G way. Think you might know it already? Well, there's always more to learn.

Finally, there is Repeat, and some people think this is the hardest of all. But I will show you how to stay motivated—for life.

*Two Turns from Zero* is an ongoing empowerment system. It works for everyone, whether you're sixteen, thirty-six, or seventy-six. Even if you're at the happiest place you've ever

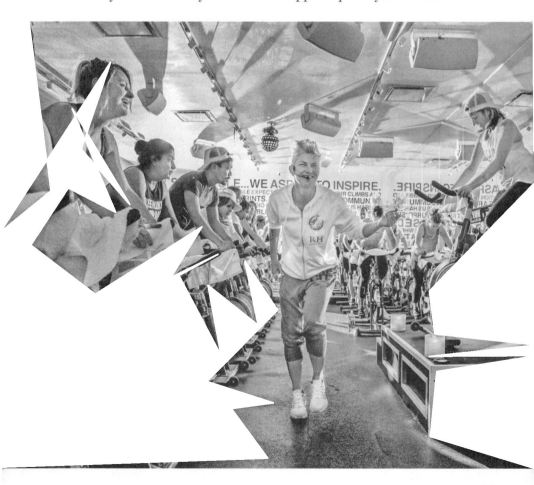

been, you can wake up tomorrow with the rainy-day blues. Or something unexpected at work can totally throw you off. Life is always full of surprises. It changes every day. Your *body* changes every day. Your goals change, your life circumstances change, and *Two Turns from Zero* is your reference guide, because today is another day to do it all over again—but this time, do it *better*. I will give you the tools to keep your body and your mind in motion, in unison, taking on life like you've never taken it on before.

Picture your most favorite place to be and imagine what it feels like to be there. I can help you make that vibration of power and contentment a major part of who you are. I say we start today.

It's only two turns from zero.

COME ON!

# PART I
# MOTIVATION

"No one
remembers
normal."

# ONE
## FINDING
## MY TRUTH

I'm *lucky*.

I had a rough childhood filled with loss, and years of self-doubt, self-medication, and addiction followed—but when I look back on those years, the first thing I tell myself is that, yes, I was really lucky. Because I *am* lucky. Every experience, tough or tender, ultimately helped me find my purpose.

People who look at me now can hardly believe that I inhaled meth on and off, sometimes every week, for years; that I drank way too much; and that I hid all this from the students I exhorted to "Be the best you can be every day." Did I listen to my own advice? Not for a long, long time.

So no, I wasn't lucky being an addict, but I was finally fortunate that I met someone who became my wingman and got me, unknowingly at first, through to my sobriety. There's no way I could have done it on my own. That's the good part of the story, but first, let's go back nearly five decades, to where my life started.

## A LITTLE BIT ABOUT THE REAL
## SG STORY . . .

When I was born, in 1968, I came out of the womb practically swinging a tennis racquet. A natural-born athlete, I was a happy little girl who just wanted to play, play, play, and who never stopped moving until I fell into bed at night (in, not surprisingly, child's pose on my knees). I've always been toned and fit and never had any problems with my weight.

Unlike my beautiful mom. My parents divorced when I was only three, and the split was incredibly difficult for her. She worked full-time while also taking care of me. She struggled with a lot; one issue in particular was her weight. She jumped from one diet to another because nothing ever worked.

This made me aware from an early age how excruciating these weight problems were for her, and for many of her friends, and how difficult it was to find the motivation to keep trying to lose weight. I was also aware that people were constantly making fun of her—sometimes directly and other

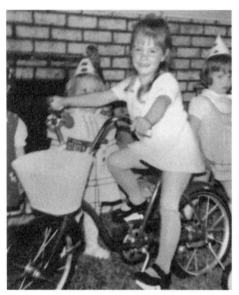

Born on the bike, age four

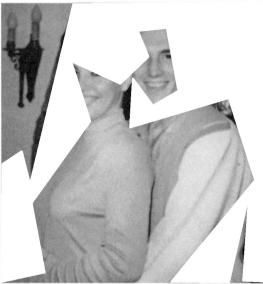

Mom and Dad

times behind her back—which caused my mom and me both to be filled with shame and hurt.

My mom was so self-conscious about her weight that the only time she would go swimming—which she loved—was at night, when there were only a few people in the pool in our apartment complex. I vividly remember watching her enter the water, surrounded by the inky darkness and the blue-lit silence of the empty pool, and seeing a smile light up her face as she let the water caress her sore legs. My heart ached for her.

The only benefit of experiencing her pain, however, is the knowledge it gave me for helping my students who are also

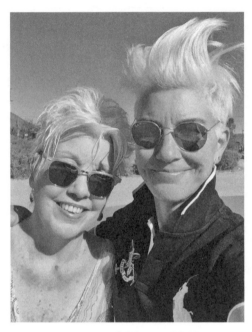

Me and Mom, 2015

struggling with weight loss. I have such deep compassion for plus-size people, because I was raised by one. I will always call my mom my hero for never letting her weight affect who she was toward me. She was a very sweet and compassionate mother, full of unconditional love for her "unique" daughter, and for that, I also feel lucky. She taught me the art of the mush—how to be a softy!

When I was eight years old, my mom nearly died in a car crash in San Jose, California, where we were living at the time, and she ended up in the same hospital where, as it happens, my grandfather was being treated for lung cancer. My father, who was by then happily remarried and busy raising his new family, only saw me every other weekend, which was what their divorce settlement decreed, so I moved in for a short time with the Harveys, my best friend's family.

They were a close-knit and devout Mormon family of eight, and some of the most amazing people I can remember from my childhood. They knew I had already been baptized into their faith the year before. That had taken place thanks to one of my friends, Dion, the son of my grandmother's neighbors up in the mountains of Calaveras County in Northern California.

I would ride my dirt bike over to Dion's house, dodging the rattlesnakes on the trails, and hang out there all day. His family was devoutly Mormon, and one Saturday when I rode over there, they told me they wanted to take me to be baptized at Lake Mont Pines. I had no idea what a baptism was, so I asked Dion what it meant, and he said you had to open your heart to God. And I thought, *Okay, my heart is open*.

"Don't be scared," he added, "because they make you walk into the lake waist deep, but with your clothes still on." I didn't understand why he was telling me not to be scared, because getting dunked sounded like a whole lot of fun! On baptism day, we walked in a line, waist deep into the lake as Dion said we would; the water was warm from the summer heat. While we stood there, we heard a short sermon from the Mormon church member who was officiating, and then he asked me to give my life to Jesus. He laid me back and I got dunked in the water, and that was it. I was baptized. The entire experience was pleasant and peaceful. The only hope I had was that, when I was dunked under the water, I could come up and be a different girl. I *was* different, in fact—I became a lot calmer. I felt like the Mormons had my back—that someone was going to save me if I died, and it was one less thing to have to think about!

Anyway, the Harveys took me in after my mother's accident, and prayed with me in the center of a circle every morning and every night, and I truly believe that their faith saved my mom, whose prognosis had been dire. I didn't really consider myself a true Mormon because my parents weren't and I wasn't that interested in churchgoing, but I was grateful for the Harveys' love and concern. My mom remained in intensive care for twenty-nine days. She was lucky to be alive, and she would live her new life as a slightly handicapped person, unable to do certain things, but she was still alive, and she was still my mom. And this was one of the first times in my life when I felt I was *lucky*.

After six weeks with the Harveys, I went to stay with my maternal grandparents, but my grandfather died about a month later. It was brutal to come home one evening from my dad's to have a lot of people over. I asked, "Where's Grandpa?" only to have my mom bring me to my room to tell me he was in heaven. I don't recall anything else from that night—just how much my throat started hurting in the middle, and how my mom's mascara ran down her cheeks from crying. I stayed with my grandmother for four more years—my mom joined us once she got out of the hospital—and then, when I was twelve, my grandmother, mom, and I moved to a different apartment complex; my grandmother got her own small apartment and my mom and I got one of our own. I still spent time with my dad, every other weekend, and every summer I went to stay with my paternal grandma, Stella.

Grandma Stella was a real go-getter. She never let having only a sixth-grade education stop her—she became a self-made millionaire. She's my main hero in life. She taught me that if you put your mind and soul into whatever you want, you *can* accomplish it, no matter what your origins are.

She wanted me to succeed more than anyone, and she also had the financial means to help me do whatever schooling I wanted. She always reminded me that when it came to school, she would pay for anything. I guess I'm glad she didn't know how much I actually hated school in those days. I think that would have broken her heart, because she loved telling me how smart she knew I was.

Grandma Stella was born in 1919 and had to drop out of school to take care of her sisters and her mom, who had tuberculosis. The family owned a restaurant, so Grandma not only had to look after her siblings and a sick mom, but she had to help run the restaurant, too. When she moved to the mountains of Calaveras County, she went to beauty school and became a hairdresser.

---

**SG TRUTH** I learned from Stella that sometimes you achieve things in life by taking a path that's different from the one you were originally going down. She never imagined she would sell real estate, and it ended up being a success story during her most tragic time after losing her best friend. Silver linings for sure, and that was how Stella lived her life.

---

Her best friend, Liz, and Liz's husband were in real estate, and when they decided to open an office, Liz told Stella that they'd bought a two-room cabin—one room for the real estate office and one room for Stella's beauty parlor. The week before they were supposed to open, Liz was killed in a logging truck accident. Bereft and despairing, Liz's husband told Stella to get her real estate license, because that was the only way to keep the business going and stay in the house. So that's what Stella did. She sold real estate for fifty years, and at her peak, she owned ten houses herself.

Grandma Stella treated me like I was an adult from the time I was a baby. She emphasized that I needed to be successful all on my own. She said I needed to have a career and to use my smarts, and to have a strong work ethic. She taught me how to drive when I was only ten.

I have to admit that Grandma Stella did drink too much—you could say it's the family curse. When she'd had too much, I was able to convince her to let me drive us home in our orange Subaru with a stick shift. But I was twelve years old at the time!

Still, even with two parents who loved me, and with Grandma Stella taking care of me in the summers, for the next four years, I felt so much imbalance in my life at home. My mom was working such incredibly long hours that by the time she got home, she was so exhausted from her day she couldn't really help me with the schoolwork I struggled with. Some nights, I would end up staying the night at a babysitter's house, or a best friend's house, which seemed fine at the time, but looking back, wasn't so great for my learning process—or getting me past my dislike of schoolwork, period. The only positive thing to come out of this imbalance was that, over the

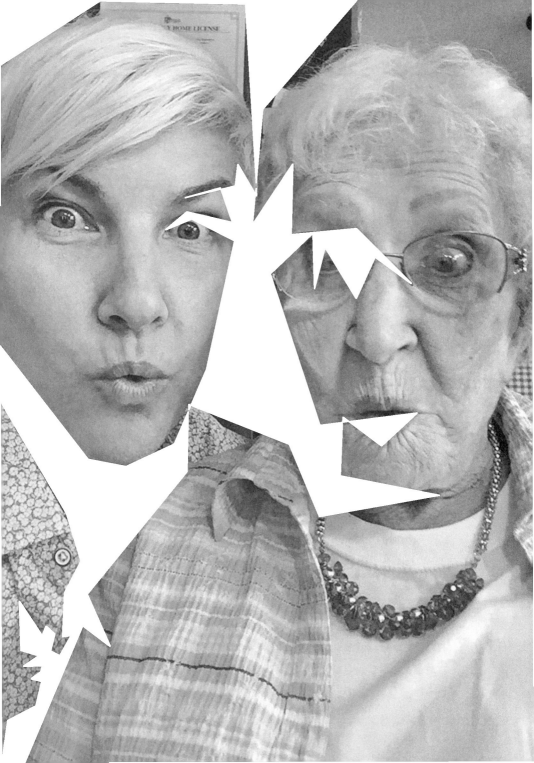

years, it helped me become a highly adaptable person who can fit into new and different environments with ease.

I'm literally happy staying anywhere, with anyone who is nice. I realize now that these childhood experiences have actually helped me embrace all kinds of people and help them feel at ease with me—which is crucial when I'm asking them to trust me in changing their lives. I know people who, as children, never had to leave their comfort zones—and that of course can be wonderful—but I can tell they have a very hard time adapting to circumstances that seem strange to them, and they have trouble sleeping in places that are unfamiliar to them. I know this seems like a quirky silver lining from my childhood—but *nothing* rattles me when it comes to sleep. I can literally sleep under a table and wake up refreshed and raring to go.

It was also during this unsettling period of my childhood that I discovered something that never left me: my own body. As I grew older, I began to feel strong and confident physically, and I became even more connected to my own physicality. What started as a survival technique eventually became my true calling as I learned how to connect the body to the mind.

"I discovered something that never left me: my own body."

This is one of the many reasons I know anyone can become an "athlete." It's an attitude as well as a physical characteristic. As soon as you start thinking about your body as your constant, faithful companion, there for you no matter what, it will give you pleasure and reassurance if you treat it right. Athletes compete . . . and this can be your attitude if you want it to be. . . .

As I hit puberty, I knew I wasn't like the other girls, and for the first time, I became uncomfortable in my own skin. It was one thing to be a tomboy, and quite another at age twelve to begin to realize that I liked other girls. I was also a teenager in the 1980s, when homophobia was still rampant, especially in my community, and the AIDS epidemic was just starting to take hold. There were signals all over the place that let me know I should keep my sexuality to myself. As early as the fourth grade, I'd been teased unmercifully by boys in my class who called me a dyke. I wasn't even sure what that meant, so I asked the playground lady, and she told me that a dyke was a girl who loved girls.

That was confusing to me, and I naively told her, "But I *do* like girls. And I want to kiss them!"

"Well," she replied with a frown, "you are not supposed to like or kiss girls."

I looked at her and willed the tears not to fall, and then ran away.

But what she said stayed with me: *It wasn't right to like girls.* So I tried to pretend my feelings away. I would play the role of a "girl," except I could be a tomboy girl—because being really good at sports was much more acceptable than being gay. Of course, this didn't get me very far, because I was never *not* gay. And as I got older, I knew I was a girl who wanted to kiss other girls.

While I was trying to work that out in my head, I plunged myself into sports, which was my form of exercise when I was a teenager. This gave me a way to be strong in my body, and that was how I created the emotional strength I needed so badly back then. Becoming stronger through sports became a way for me to handle the emotional pain I was experiencing, and team sports kept me going through middle school.

All eighth graders had electives, but that's where things got doubly complicated for me. When it was time to do the choosing, the boys got to pick "Boys Sports," which meant running, basketball, and volleyball. Sounds good, right? But when it came time for the girls to choose, here's the choice we had: Home Economics. So much for choices, right?

I guess I was bolder in those days than I wanted to give myself credit for, because I asked to be put with the boys. I could see they were actually being given choices—and I wanted to do those sports. The school said no, but I kept pushing, and when I got my parents to sign off on it, they finally gave in.

Well, once I was in, nine other girls followed me—no big surprise!—and that was the end of the "Boys Sports" class. Thanks to me, the name "Boys Sports" turned into just "Sports"—which is what it should have been in the first place.

In high school, sports ruled my life. I had become a superstar athlete. My coaches loved me—so did my teachers, even though they were still frustrated by my endless doodling and daydreaming and chatty ways. I have to admit it: I was a classic flake girl who never turned in homework on time and never studied for any tests. The only thing that got me in the school door every day was team sports, because I just didn't go for the books and studying part.

It's true that sometimes I got benched for a few games during the season because my grades were so bad, but I still refused to do the work. During my sophomore year, my mother and I moved to a different neighborhood, and that meant a different school. The new administration hadn't yet figured out how lazy I was academically, but they were thrilled to have me playing on their sports teams.

The big eye-opener for me at that school was that I met a lot of other gay kids, and that helped me to finally come out. These friends supported me, and I fell in love with one of them. Finally, I felt real love.

That was a really great thing to be introduced to, but along with that came introductions to some very best new friends: alcohol and marijuana.

It seemed that whenever I'd be hanging out with my friends, we'd drink beer, wine, and those berry-colored wine coolers. I'd already started smoking pot at my old school, but I smoked more frequently at this new school. And getting high every day helped me deal with how much I hated my schoolwork.

I remember being high when I went to tryouts for junior varsity basketball. Even the possibility that I might jeopardize my placement on the team wasn't enough to make me stop lighting up in those days. I'll never forget the day they released the team roster. I scanned up and down the list. No matter how hard I looked, I couldn't find my name. I practically panicked. What had I done? Had my habit botched the tryout? People around me started laughing at my reaction. The reason I couldn't find my name on the *junior* varsity list was that I was already so advanced as a player that I'd been placed on the *varsity* team. That was unheard of for a freshman!

That was a real ego boost for a fourteen-year-old, and it felt great, but the other thing it did was make me feel indestructible. So what was a little pot smoking every day? It didn't stop me from making the varsity basketball team. I was a *star*. I was invincible. I was also taking my first steps on a very tough road that nearly led me to ruin. Oh, how I wish I could go back to that fourteen-year-old and tell her what I know today!

Things got even crazier when I went back to my old high school for my senior year. I wanted to switch because their basketball team was better, and I also had a new girlfriend and wanted to be closer to where she lived. The season was going great, and I was the highest scorer in the league, until suddenly I got a devastating knee injury. I had to have surgery, and I was completely out of commission.

Around this time, my mom—who was so devoted to our basketball team that she was voted "Mom of the Year"—was going through some really tough times financially, which, understandably, had left her preoccupied and stressed and not able to focus as much on what was going on with me. So with no diploma and no job, I dropped out of high school and followed my girlfriend, who had a volleyball college scholarship at California Polytechnic, San Luis Obispo.

Now what was I going do? I got a job at a summer camp at the local YMCA in San Luis Obispo. Somehow I thought it was easier to just bail on my life and escape into adulthood than it was to finish high school as an eighteen-year-old gay person. All I wanted at that time was peace and employment. The YMCA was a sanctuary that offered love and acceptance—and most of all, a job! I led camps and after-school programs, worked in the actual gym, and taught racquetball. I started playing so much racquetball that I became the 1986 novice champion for central California.

And then one day, fate intervened: One of the fitness instructors wasn't able to make it to teach her abs class, and one of the students—who knew I was an athlete and figured I was capable of training everyone at the gym—asked if I would teach the class. I said yes, and it was as if I discovered by accident exactly what I was always supposed to be doing. Teaching other people how to exercise correctly felt as natural as breathing, and I was instantly hooked. For the first time, I discovered how great it felt to make other people feel good about their bodies. And even better, that experience gave me as much back as I got from the killer workouts I did for my own body.

That's how my career as a fitness coach and trainer began.

When my girlfriend graduated, she wanted to move back to the San Jose area, and I didn't. At this time, I was having problems getting along with my parents, and she had not told her parents that she was a lesbian. Her parents were devoutly Catholic, and we had told them we were just roommates. We even went to church with them three times a week.

After I struggled a bit over the what, where, when, and how to manage my life, I knew I could count on Grandma Stella to come to the rescue. She actually made me move in with her, go back to school, and get my high school diploma. She even wanted me to practice real estate with her, which I just couldn't do, but I did decide she was right about school, and I was proud to have that high school diploma.

I was still living with Grandma Stella and wondering what was next when a dear friend, who I have to keep nameless here, got "saved" at a megachurch in Torrance, California, and decided she was straight after telling me she'd thought she was gay. She wanted a family and thought it would never happen if she were ever to be living with a woman—this was in 1990, mind you, when it was very, very rare for a gay couple to have children. Another friend took her to the church, not because he thought it would convince her to be straight, but because he wanted her to have some religion in her life, and knew she was struggling with issues of spirituality.

She found the experience so amazing that she asked me to go to church with her. I happily agreed. Despite my Mormon baptism, I considered myself a Christian but not affiliated with any denomination. I was simply open to every religion and didn't have any judgment about any of them—I thought of myself as a spiritual person who liked to pray occasionally, but religion was not at the top of my priority list.

So we went to the Cottonwood Christian Center, and I got saved again, this time by Pastor Bayless Conley. And it was on television. I got up in front of two thousand people and professed my love to God. And the weirdest thing was that I literally got lifted out of that freaking seat by God. I'm not kidding! I don't even know how to describe the sensation—I just know that I must have been meant to experience it. I really feel as though I was blessed by this congregation for life.

Afterward, we were taken off the stage so that they could explain what had just taken place, and one elderly woman pulled me aside. She was so sweet, and I had no idea who she was.

"My child," she said, "you're such a beautiful girl. Jesus loves you, or you would not have been chosen." She smiled beatifically. "I want to tell you something very special. I am not usually here on days with our new members of the church, but today, I felt that I had to come. You see, Pastor Bayless is my son. The man who gave the sermon and who saved you. Looking at you, my dear, makes me realize why I am here now, today, and it is so I can tell you that you are one of God's chosen ones. You really are a chosen child. This is a very, very amazing day in the eyes of the Lord."

*Well*, I mean, *come on*. To say I was astonished is a rather large understatement. I had no idea what to say or do after hearing that.

"God wants you to speak," she went on, more emphatically.

"He wants you to speak. He wants you to save lives; he has chosen you to save lives."

You have to remember, this was before I had any real teaching experience, except for some fill-ins at the YMCA.

She wasn't finished yet: "He has blessed you with a specific tongue, and I want to see if you're feeling what Jesus has planned for you in this moment. Have you ever heard of speaking in tongues?"

"Yes," I told her. I was too shy to explain that I knew about this phenomenon because I'd had a devoutly religious friend in high school, and when I spent time with her family, they often spoke about it.

"Do you think you could speak right now?" the woman asked.

I nodded, and she grabbed my hand, and I started speaking some weird language. I had no idea what I was saying. She started crying as she patted my hand. "You are chosen," she said between sobs. "I want you to know how special you are. This will be one of the most memorable days of your life because the Lord has saved you. And you are to speak about Jesus."

When I told my gay-friend-who-didn't-want-to-be-gay-anymore about this conversation, I was torn. Clearly, something profound *had* happened, and I *had* been chosen, but I didn't want to do what Pastor Bayless's mom wanted me to do—to give up the life I was living and devote it to Jesus. I still liked to drink. I still liked to smoke pot. I still liked to party.

She nodded. "I knew it," she told me. "I knew you were the one, because I wasn't chosen like that. I can't speak that language. I've tried, but it's not my gift. That's why I wanted you to go to church with me. I just *knew*."

So I started going to this church for about six months, and moved in with a platonic guy friend who I'll call Stan. He had a large apartment in Irvine, with a huge living room in the front with a church-like ceiling. I would put on a Christian radio station and stand in the middle of the living room and worship, speaking in tongues and singing the songs and the hymns. I would open my heart to God and ask for his strength and his power, and I asked Him to please guide me. I didn't know what the fuck I was going to do with my life. I didn't know where I was going.

Surprisingly, all the time I spent praying helped me stop drinking and partying without the effort I thought it would take. Still, I honestly did not know what was next because I'd been heartbroken by another failed relationship, and it dawned on me that Stan, who was as straight as a man could be, was dropping hints that he liked me. Liked me a little too much, even though he knew I was gay.

Complicating our friendship was that he liked to come home and tell me what he was doing at work—he was starting a porn website, and this was when Internet porn was barely a thing. (Trust me—you can't make things like this up!) His sexual interest in me and his job that I couldn't respect made my living arrangement increasingly fraught.

"I'll help you," he would say to me. "I know you're on this new path. God wants you to be with a man. *I'm* your man."

But he wasn't, and I knew he never would be. So I threw myself even more fervently into trying to save people who didn't believe or weren't worshiping. Because after all, that woman at the church had said this was my gift, right? She'd said this was my purpose.

So I went around to as many of my other friends as I could, and I tried to convince them to go to church with me, but most of them looked at me as if I had two heads and said, "Stacey, you've lost your mind. . . ."

Maybe I was a bit loopy with the whole trying-to-convert-other-people thing, but I will admit that something magical happened to me during this enlightenment. It changed me forever. It gave me that feeling that someone truly believed in me. Pastor Bayless's mom told me that God believed in me . . . and I believed her, and I believed *Him*. That meant I was worth something. Someone finally believed in me, believed I was meant to heal people.

Then one night, something amazing happened. I was lying in my bed. I had prayed most of the day, and I was praying again, and suddenly I felt like I was levitating off the bed. *Oh my God, what is happening to me?* It was as if my chest opened up, and I swear I saw this imaginary hand come down—it was God's hand, I knew it—and it came down and pushed hard on my chest because I had so much anxiety about what I was going to do . . . and He just put His hand on my heart and told me that everything was going to be fine, and the pressure of His hand was so comforting I fell asleep.

---

SG TRUTH   For several years, I was out of communication with my family. I didn't visit anyone, or even check in to see how they were. From the time I was eighteen, I would say I was "on the run" until I went to Grandma Stella's. After that, I *still* was not so great at being a great daughter; it wasn't until I got sober years later that I was able to be present and helpful to my entire family.

---

When I woke up the next morning, I knew it was time to go. Time to make a big change in what I was going to do with the rest of my life. Time to say good-bye to that apartment and my friends. Way past time to get away from Stan. Amazingly enough, a few hours later, I got a call from my friend Barry. "Hey, Nosh," she said—she called me Nosh because I loved to nosh on bagels—"what are you up to? I'm moving to LA to start a PR company. Do you wanna come work with me? I'll pay you. You need to get out of there."

That was the clincher. I moved up to Los Angeles in 1991. My own Sin City. I ditched church, and I started doing stand-up comedy. I took classes at the Improv and did so well at my showcase that I got an agent who was really interested in developing me as a comedic actress—this was the same time Ellen DeGeneres was big on the circuit. The problem became me choosing the night life over the professional "comic" life. I made the choice to get in with the wrong crowd, and started partying and doing drugs again.

The good news in the bad news was that these party people were also, paradoxically, very healthy. They were totally into eating right and fitness. And speaking of fitness, this is when I first heard about this thing they called Spinning—they were *obsessed* with it. They literally did not stop talking about it. I remember being impressed that they didn't seem to care if they had to spend more than an hour in traffic on the 405 Freeway if it meant they would end up at their favorite Spinning class.

Finally, after I'd been hearing so much about it, I had to try it right away. I loved it! I was hooked. After the first class, I wanted to be the one picking the music; after the third class, I knew what I really wanted was to lead the entire thing, and I was determined to become an instructor.

Okay, here's where I have to admit something. I had to tell a lie to get my first real Spin-instructor job. The job was at the Workout Warehouse, which at the time was the hottest, celebrity-heavy studio in West Hollywood, and the only one that had Spin classes. It was run by Doug and Cheo, two big muscle-heads and beautiful gay guys who welcomed everyone to all their classes.

I told myself that claiming to have taught my own classes wasn't that bad of a lie because I had such good intentions and was so desperate for the job. (Um, *sorry*, it was still a lie!) I asked a friend who ran a much-smaller fitness studio where

I had started taking classes if he would cover for me and say I taught there even though I didn't. He knew that once I'd taken over an aerobics class when one of the instructors hadn't shown, and a lot of people told me I'd held down a pretty good I've-done-this-before kind of attitude as I led that one class. He shrugged and said no problem.

So I lied on my application about my experience teaching Spin classes, and was very lucky that Doug and Cheo didn't thoroughly vet my résumé, or I would have been busted. I got the job. I was a really awful instructor at first, thanks in part to the antiquainted microphone technology at the time. This was before cordless microphones were invented, so I had to hold the mike in my hand and talk and spin and do my thing. I was good at the doing-my-thing part of teaching from day one, but it took me a while to get used riding the bike and holding the mike so I could talk and teach and check on my students' form at the same time.

I owe a lot to Doug and Cheo. They taught me how to teach the method that I teach now. I learned how to put musicality and physicality together on the bike, and to do a lot of pushups, a lot of turning and burning, and a lot of weight training on the bike. In fact, I owe my career to their kindness and their smarts.

It wasn't long before I became very successful as an instructor. I thought I was doing awesomely well. My classes were written up in magazines and featured on *The Rosie O'Donnell Show*. My career seemed to be really taking off. I was working at one of LA's most famous fitness studios, and I was regularly having eighty people take each of my Spin classes. A lot of people in my classes were well-known celebrities, and some of them became my friends. And outside of my classes, I was partying more and more. Did my fitness clients know that I was also a partier? Some did, some didn't. Did they care? Not a bit. My coworkers didn't care, either—because they were partiers, too.

This was the 1990s, in Los Angeles, and nearly everybody (well, not *everybody*, but *most*) in the fitness industry was on either cocaine, meth, ketamine, or Ecstasy. And sometimes all of the above. We were living the Hollywood life, baby.

Everyone in my circle was doing drugs all the time, and that's all I needed to know for me to think it was all okay for me to do it, too. I loved being high. It was how I made myself feel less anxious and how I shielded myself from the pain in the world that I was unable to face.

I knew going in to all this that alcoholism ran in my family, and it was something I would have to battle with myself. But even as much as I knew this, I plunged feetfirst into this decade. I wasn't just an occasional drug user and pot smoker and someone who liked to drink. I was someone who *had* to use. Looking back at this time of my life is where I realize that I crossed the line and became an addict. A functioning one . . . one who could show up to work high, lie about it, and know that people literally had no clue. I occasionally run into people now who knew me during this decade, and they still can't believe it when I tell them what was going on back then. That's how good I was at hiding the truth from nearly everyone—especially myself.

I am not being glib when I say I was very much a "functioning addict," because I was still an athlete, and still fit and healthy, which meant I could party until late at night, and still show up for work the next morning, ready to lead a kick-ass Spin class, as if I'd gone to bed at nine P.M. and slept like a baby through the night. Although I must admit that sometimes I did sleep through classes, and got fired many times. But I was so good at teaching that I always got hired back!

I don't want to give the impression that while I leading this partying lifestyle I was *unhappy*. A lot of the time, it was amazing. I had an unbelievably good time. And that's one of the reasons I stayed addicted so long. I was having such a great time, so why stop the party? So what if it's three A.M., and I have a one-on-one training session at six A.M., and I'm teaching a class at seven thirty A.M.? No problem. I can do it. Do it all and bring it on, 100 percent. Oy.

It's amazing that I didn't even sober up when a terrible tragedy took place in 1999. Seann, my half brother from my dad's second marriage, was living in Hawaii at the time. He was twenty-three years old, and his girlfriend had lost a baby who was stillborn. Not long after that, he and five of his friends were driving in a car when they hit a patch of water and hydroplaned on the freeway. The car flipped, everyone got ejected, and they all lived. Everyone except Seann. My little brother was the only one who died, and he was the only one wearing his seat belt.

It hit me very hard, but I pretended it didn't. About a month after his death, I got a strange feeling that I should go out clubbing on a night I usually wouldn't go out. I didn't want to, but this feeling was so overwhelming that I finally gave in. I decided to go to a private underground bar I'd been invited to before but hadn't yet been. A few minutes after I arrived, a group of young straight kids came up to me and said, "Are you Seann Griffith's sister?" I said I was, and one of the girls said, "I was with him just before he died."

I stared at her for a moment, stunned. I'd never met those kids before, and I still don't know how they got in there. And then it hit me. *My brother sent them.* "He was so happy," this girl went on. "We can't believe he's gone. He was the love of our community."

We all sat down in one of those weird Kumbaya moments, with our arms around one another as we all started to cry in the middle of the club. It was like a sign—of something special, because I never got a chance to say good-bye to my brother. He was such a happy guy, and he made a lot of other people happy with his spirit.

I remember that he used call me on the phone, and he would say, "*Dude,* I met someone who knows you. Can you believe it?" He was fascinated that people he met would actually know his big sister.

A few days after that night at the bar, I went to a party with some friends. All of us were either fitness trainers or actors, and we all were making it in our careers at the same time. I had started doing a TV show that was on the Travel Channel called *Intersection*. (Please do *not* google that one, as it's embarrassingly bad!) My classes were doing great. Two of my students from this circle had been on *Beverly Hills 90210*, which had recently gone off the air. Christian Kane had his band, Kane, and was shooting *Life or Something Like It* with Angelina Jolie. Vin Diesel had shot *The Fast and the Furious* during this time, and I remember standing in the kitchen with my friend Lee, who introduced me to Vin, who said, pointing to Vin with a wide smile, "See him, Stacey? This guy's about to blow up. Everyone in this house has blown up. It's a good-luck house."

A psychic had been hired for the party that night. I sat down with her, and she said, "What do you want me to read you for?" and I said, "My brother, Seann."

She closed her eyes and said, "Wow, I just got a really big flash of a rainbow. Seann's with us, and he's standing at the foot of the rainbow holding a wiener dog."

My jaw dropped. "That's our family dog that died, Heidi."

The psychic nodded. "Seann is surrounded by water. Does that make sense?"

I nodded. "Yes. He just died in Hawaii."

"He's there with the dog, and wants you to know he's okay, and he's super happy where he is."

That was a comfort.

Around this time, I'd decided to clean up my act. I cut down on the drugging and drinking. A few months later, I was actually sober and not missing the partying at all. My girlfriend of two years and I had decided that a big change was needed—in large part to help me stick to my sobriety. We had decided together that we had a major problem with using and drinking—that was an understatement!—and we finally needed to take control of our lives.

We managed to quit cold turkey (I have never been to rehab); we did this together successfully and started to think of ways to get out of LA. I was offered an amazing job in Atlanta, to be the group fitness director for a gym chain. We discussed having kids. We ended the lease on our LA apartment and bought a small house in Atlanta. I put every single piece of my life on a moving truck. Then, the night before we were going to leave, my girlfriend did something so unexpected and so devastating to me (I can't share the details) that we split up. I'm sure in hindsight we were both equally responsible for the behavior that led up to this moment, but needless to say, we ended a potentially great future at the time.

Shattered, I asked a very close friend of mine, whom I will call Michael, if I could temporarily move into one of his spare bedrooms. He said sure. (Remember, I have no problem being bounced around, moving, or being in a new environment.)

Michael was one of my students in the front row in my Spinning classes at the Workout Warehouse. If I played any song recorded before 1980, he would get up and leave. I'd be like, "Hey, Michael, I'm playing Hall and Oates now, bye!" and everyone else would say, "Bye, Michael!" as he got off his bike in a huff and stomped out. He just hated vintage music—it reminded him of each of the three wives he had married and then divorced. He'd always known he was gay, but he hadn't wanted to admit it. He didn't want his ex-wives to know. He didn't want hardly *anyone* to know, in fact, and he trusted me to keep his secret private.

Michael and I became incredibly close. We nurtured each other, and we adored each other. There was only one problem: He was much further entrenched in the world of drugs than I had ever been, and he introduced me to meth. He'd made enough money in his career to finance his habit, and he was totally into it. A lot of gay men in Hollywood in the 1990s were into it. I remember being scared to death of it at first, because Michael smoked it, and I knew that inhaling the drug was so, so bad and a guarantee of a much quicker, full-blown addiction. I also knew enough about addicts to understand how smoking drugs versus smoking cigarettes was not in the same stratosphere . . . let's just be clear! I stopped being scared once I started putting it up my nose. I'd snort it, he'd smoke it, and finally it got to the point where, as a joke, he would blow it in my face, and then in my mouth. I was just fooling myself.

I knew if I touched that pipe, my meth addiction would become a huge problem. But because the drug was so addictive, I was soon smoking meth even after swearing I never would. Lying to yourself is something addicts do. I'd become living proof of that cliché "slippery slope" everyone talks about—but at that point, it wasn't just talk, it was my life. I remember it being like your first taste of sugar as a kid . . . just as bad, and all you think about is wanting *more*.

Ironically, one of the reasons I'd been using drugs all along was as self-medication. They helped me avoid my problems and frustrations, and took me out of my challenging life situations. But meth was something completely different. My meth high paradoxically made me feel *normal*. Focused. I am not hedging when I say that I got so much done when I was on meth. (I learned years later that meth and Adderall both affect the same neurotransmitters in your brain, and as I have ADHD, meth functioned in much the same way as the prescription med. Which is scary!)

As I had earlier in my LA years, I thought of myself as a fully functioning addict who was fully in control. Crazy, yes, but that's how addicts defend their addiction. I tried not to miss a class I was teaching. I worked incredibly hard. I became totally obsessed with my cleanliness. I had enough beauty products in my bathroom to rival Sephora. I took vitamins. I ate well. I trained every day. I was sleeping more. What's so insane is that this became my new normal.

Michael was a functioning addict, too. All this time, he was able to work as hard as I did and was successful at his business. No one outside of our circle would ever have had a clue that meth was a part of our lives. I was so focused during this time that I went to sound engineering school and was able to research music for hours in between the Spin classes I taught. I was also able to keep up with my personal training clients as well as my own workouts. Soon, I even had a second career as a DJ.

This crazy lifestyle went on for three years.

Then, I fell in love again, and that made me want to stop doing meth. This girlfriend did not like the idea of the drugs at
all, so I had to make a choice. It had really gotten to the point
where drugs had taken control of my life . . . so I managed to
kick my addiction cold turkey again and moved out of Michael's (but I kept my room there just in case). Michael wasn't
so lucky—he continued on that same dark path, all by himself.
At least when we were living together, I seemed to have had a
moderating effect on him. I was guilt-ridden leaving him alone
in that apartment, but I knew I had to try to change my life.

It also didn't help that his boyfriend, whom he was passion-
ately in love with, broke up with him and moved away. Plus,
Michael had a painful genetic neuropathic condition that
made it hard for him to get out of bed in the morning, and his
drug abuse only made it worse. He often talked almost sar-
castically about committing suicide—it was very hard to tell
with him, given his sharp and dark sense of humor—and he
had made a few halfhearted attempts that his friends and I
thought were more a cry for help than any real determination
to do it. This had happened enough that we never took him as
seriously as we should have.

I knew Michael was in a bad way, but I was shocked when one
day he told me that he had gotten a euthanasia kit from some
sketchy online site. I panicked and called all of our friends
and told them that Michael was serious this time. I said they
needed to get right over to his house, but they didn't believe
me and thought he was just trying to get attention, even as I

begged and pleaded and told them there was a real euthanasia kit in his room. Only one of my friends came over, and he talked to Michael for a long time, and on the way out told me there was *no way* he was serious.

I went into his room, and Michael was lying on his bed. I sat down next to him and told him I was calling the police. It wasn't the first time I'd made that threat.

"Why would you do that?" he said. "If you do, I'll ruin your career. I'll call the gym where you love your job and tell them you're a drug addict. I'll *ruin* you. For real. You cannot get in my way. If you love me, let me go. I just want to go. Remember when you used to go with me to the convalescent home to see my father? Do you remember how awful that was for me, how my father suffered? I don't want to end up like that. I don't want you or anyone else to have to do that for me. I just want to go now. Let me go, okay?"

It wasn't okay, of course. I pleaded with him. I begged. I sobbed. I threatened to call the police again, my job be damned. "What can I do to make you stay here?" I asked. "Do you want me to move back? Do you want to go to rehab?"

"Well," he said, "you can have sex with me."

That actually made me laugh. "Shut up!" I said.

"No, I'm serious. I'll stay alive if you have sex with me."

I looked at him. "I'm not doing that, Michael," I told him. "I don't sleep with people just to get what I want. You know that. It's not the type of person I am. Don't do this to me."

Michael smiled. He knew how much I loved him as a friend,

and he also knew I could not have sex with him. He would have taken care of me forever, would have given me anything I wanted; but he knew I wouldn't do it. And I knew he was proud of me, in that moment, for staying true to myself.

So then I tried to turn the tables on him. "Let me see if it works," I said, grabbing the euthanasia kit. "Let's try it on me first."

No way would I have done it, but I wanted to scare some sense into Michael.

"Don't touch that thing," he said. "What, are you *crazy*?"

"No, but how do you think I feel, listening to you talk like this?"

Michael leaned back and sighed. "Look, Stacey, you have a whole life to live, an entire career, and so much to look forward to. But please promise me a few things. I promise you from the other side"—that's what we called it—"I promise that when I get to the other side, I will watch over you, I will guide you. I will take care of everything. However I can guide you, I will."

Tears were sliding down my cheeks.

"But you've got to *stop*," he went on. "I mean it. You've got to stop doing drugs, you have to stop smoking, and you have to stop drinking."

"Oh, gee, that sounds fun," I said, trying to be flip.

Michael ignored me. "When you do that, all those things, I promise I'll totally take care of you," he said again.

We stayed up late talking. In the morning, I left because his sister and brother-in-law came over to see how he was doing and keep him company. As I was walking out the door, I said good-bye to him. For the last time.

His last words to me were: "See you on the other side. . . ."

I'm not sure what words were exchanged between Michael and his family. They obviously weren't strong enough to make the impact he needed to change his mind. At this point in his life I don't think anyone could have changed his mind. He was on a mission to leave. . . .

After he was gone, I went off the deep end. No matter how much I told myself that Michael had truly wanted to die, I was tortured by guilt and self-recriminations, and my only way of dealing with that was to do drugs even more often. I felt that I was lost without him. We had spent an enormous amount of time together. He had been like a surrogate dad, a brother, a boyfriend (without the sex). He was like my main squeeze.

Our plan was to be in each other's lives forever. But so many other things were happening for Michael. He was beginning to feel his age, and in West Hollywood, where there are so many hot young men running around and you're the old guy who feels like a dinosaur, it got to his ego. Michael was also having a lot of financial problems. His life wasn't going the way he expected, and I think he just couldn't cope anymore. I honestly think he died of a broken heart. He just gave up.

I felt like part of me nearly did, too.

The next year was pure hell. I missed Michael desperately. I felt him near me, every day (and still do). I talked to him a *lot*. I had his initials inked on my right calf. Having these conversations was like a soul-soothing meditation, but it wasn't enough. Michael had committed suicide in one desperate moment, but I was doing it slowly, by degrees, every time I took another hit. On the outside, I was the glowing California girl, brimming with health and vitality, a superstar Spin instructor with famous friends and a fabulous lifestyle. On the inside, I was going down.

I knew I had to find a way to quit, and it wasn't going to be easy. It took quite some time of me dealing with some hard truths about myself, of spending the time I needed to try to understand myself better, and many weeks of couch-surfing and staying in friends' guesthouses (there were two; very LA!) when I knew I had to pull it together, some way, somehow. I'm not an Alcoholics Anonymous type, and I'm not the rehab-going kind of gal, so I just kept reading spiritual books, praying to Michael to help me from wherever he was, praying to my grandparents, praying to all the friends I had lost over the years . . . to help me.

"I am living proof that you can recover and detoxify and cleanse and clear."

How did I do it, finally? I fell in love with an incredible woman, a normal family person with children, and I knew that you cannot be on drugs or have drugs in your life if you want to be a good partner.

She was the most amazing mother, and it was clear early on that if I wanted to be with her, I had to clean up my act. My therapist says that at first you quit for someone else, and then eventually your training wheels fall off, and you're riding the sober bike all for yourself. And that's exactly what happened.

I do have to admit that for the first six years of our relationship, I lied about how bad my addiction had really been. I just didn't want her to know what I'd done. I was full of shame and guilt, and was really embarrassed to tell her how bad it was. And I kept drinking for the first two years we were together. I got really drunk at a fortieth birthday party, and we got in a fight, and she told me that if I ever had one more drink, she would not be with me anymore. Period. My behavior that night was reprehensible.

So I stopped. And with her help, I conquered my drug addiction and my alcoholism. This wasn't easy, because as I said earlier, almost everyone in my family is an alcoholic. Even Grandma Stella, who's ninety-seven years old, still loves her martinis. Who am I to tell her that alcohol is bad for your health? It wasn't bad for *hers*. She's beautiful, and healthy, and looks amazing!

At first, I missed the friends I'd had and the clubbing lifestyle that went with my addictions. But I don't miss it now. I love my sober life. I love who I am as a person more than I loved that person who partied. Sobriety has become such a big part of who I am that I identify more as a sober person than I did as a functioning addict.

I went from calling it partying, which sounds like so much fun, to admitting I was an addict, which is really no fun at all and negatively affects those around you, not to mention your-self. Now I can say out loud that I lied to myself about being an addict and that I had been lying to myself for a long time. But I had to own it. When I finally did that, it was my first real step into my recovery.

All my years of addiction, and all my experiences in life, are a huge part of why I am as successful as I am as a teacher. I didn't just magically end up where I am today. The climb and the struggle were fucking brutal. It was more than twenty years of climbing and never giving up. Having experienced that myself is why I can help people go from the bottom to the top. I know what it's like because I've really been there and I've really done that.

I am living proof that you can recover and detoxify and cleanse and clear and become a totally different person. I am not proud of a lot of the choices I made. Many of them were horrendous. But I am here to say that you *can* rise from the depths of it. One second at a time.

And find your purpose, as I found mine.

"Figuring out
your purposes
is a process."

# TWO
# THE POWER
# OF PURPOSE

When you are working within your purpose, it is much easier to live in your Ultimate Center. Purpose is what allows you to stay strong emotionally and physically in the face of adversity, and provides intrinsic motivation to all that you do.

Figuring out your life purpose is one of the most important discoveries you'll ever have. Some people know what it is when they're children; they declare that they're going to be a doctor or a teacher or an astronaut or a carpenter or an artist, and don't waver in their path. Others are not so sure, and graduate from high school or college and still don't know. It takes years of doing different jobs to find out what they're best at. Others realize that their life purpose is being a good parent or a good friend, or giving back to their community.

I overcame enormous obstacles on my journey toward figuring myself out and fine-tuning my purpose. Michael's death was the tipping point. I knew he was right. I knew I had to shape up or die. I had to turn that knob way, *way* away from zero to get *control* over myself and move on to better things.

How can you do the same?

Figuring out your purpose is a process. Many people find it incredibly difficult to actually sit down with themselves and say what it is they really, truly want to be, especially if they have made life choices they didn't want to make to please other people (such as going into a particular field to please their parents or to make a lot of money).

## DON'T BE AFRAID TO ASK FOR HELP

Asking for help can be easy. You have the flu, so you ask your doctor to help you get better. You don't understand how to do math equations, so you ask your teacher for help. You don't know why your computer keeps glitching, so you ask someone smart at the computer store. Those problems aren't easy ones, but they don't involve emotions, so we aren't embarrassed to ask for help with them.

But dealing with emotional problems involves digging deep enough into what's truly going on, and many people have trouble doing that. It's too painful, or it's too daunting. To me, people who live like that are just existing, just getting by in life, without scratching beneath the surface. I find that terribly sad, because they're losing out on life without really trying.

I can say that because I felt like that, too. I wasn't able to admit to myself that I was stuck and flailing. I knew I needed help—something to give me that jolt to haul me out of my rut. It wasn't until I went to a Tony Robbins seminar that I was able to clarify just how much help I needed. He didn't pussyfoot around when he said, "If you do what you always do, you'll get what you've always gotten." That one particular statement got to me, in my gut, and I was so inspired that it made me ready to turn that knob two turns from zero before I'd even left the auditorium.

Part of Tony's rare gift, I realized later—one Oprah has as well—was his ability to connect to more than three thousand people that weekend. We all left feeling as if he'd personally sat us down, one on one, in a tiny room, and asked us how he could *help* us. Everyone was able to filter his coaching into their own personal needs at the time. That is the mark of a true healer.

Tony also made me realize that I needed much more specific help with the issues that had made me an addict. I started therapy over a decade ago, and my therapist and my partner are still who I go to now for help. I firmly believe that every human being needs therapy; it's a sign of strength to say "I need help" and have a trained and competent third party give you guidance. When you need help getting your body in shape, you go to a trainer. When you need help with your emotions, you go to a therapist. If you need help getting motivated, you buy this book. One of the reasons people love coming to my class is because I speak using the language I've learned over the years in therapy.

One of the concepts I've often discussed in therapy is the notion of being present for whatever it is you're doing. This kind of mindfulness is important when you're working out. You need to be present for yourself and not, for example, distracted by what you're reading in a magazine as you slowly pedal on a recumbent bicycle. I do my utmost to be fully *present* for my students. I always show up 100 percent alert—well, okay, let's say *90 percent* of the time, because, as you know, some days are just a little harder to gear up, for no reason other than it's just one of those days! Long gone are those days when I taught with a hangover or poisons in my body. I come shaman ready.

My years in therapy also taught me that it's the perfect place to talk about your demons and whatever is plaguing you. A good therapist will help you recognize the patterns that you click into in order to stay in your comfort zone. Only by recognizing and identifying these patterns are you able to break free of them. Just talking about things that happened to me decades ago—things that were so painful they're still stuck in my memory—is incredibly cathartic for me. I think everybody can benefit from some kind of therapy. It's not just for serious problems when times are really tough, or to treat mental illness. It's the best way that healthy people can stay that way. Going to therapy when life is good can make life even *better*.

I think a good therapist is the best kind of life coach, wanting everyone on the team to find the sweet spot and thrive under pressure. A brilliant coach gives you ideas, and then watches as a neutral third party, with kindness and empathy, but without judgment, as you implement them.

Only you know what kind of help is the right fit for you. I also have my rituals that keep me grounded. You might feel more comfortable in a house of worship; or confiding in friends whose wisdom you value, going to a mentor, reading books like this one, or doing the kind of Moving Meditation you'll read about in this book, the kind you can get in a class like mine. Whatever you choose, you have to respect and click with the person who delivers the advice you need to hear.

You can also go on YouTube and type in "How to Find My Purpose." There are more than four *million* results—talks, seminars, classes, and other videos. With help, you should be able to set up some sort of spiritual practice that refreshes your spirit and gives you the confidence to mentally process what's going on in your life and focus on your goals, dreams, and purpose.

There are lines in a spoken-word song by Baz Luhrmann called "Everybody's Free (to Wear Sunscreen)" (which was adapted from a column written by Mary Schmich in the *Chicago Tribune* in 1997): "Advice is a form of nostalgia." That really struck a chord with me, as I realized that, when working on finding your purpose, you don't want to totally wipe away the past, but to take inventory of it, to learn from it, to acknowledge the mistakes and successes, and to then move forward. If you look at yourself as constantly evolving, it's easier to unstick yourself from those habitual patterns that might be comfortable, but that are holding you back from your true purpose.

## MAP IT OUT

One of the best ways to begin to figure out your true purpose and what may be holding you back from reaching it is to create a MAP. MAP stands for Make a Plan. MAP it out. But where do you start on your MAP? At the beginning, of course. (You knew I was going to say that!)

Get a piece of paper or a notebook, and make a list of all the important areas of your life: work, relationships, friendships, financial health, physical health,

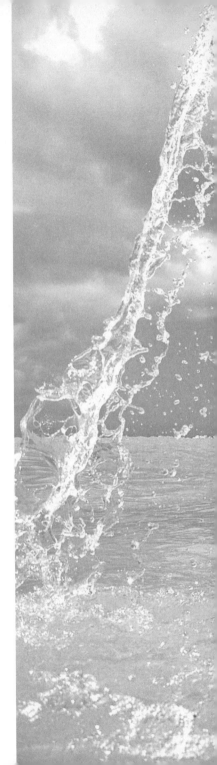

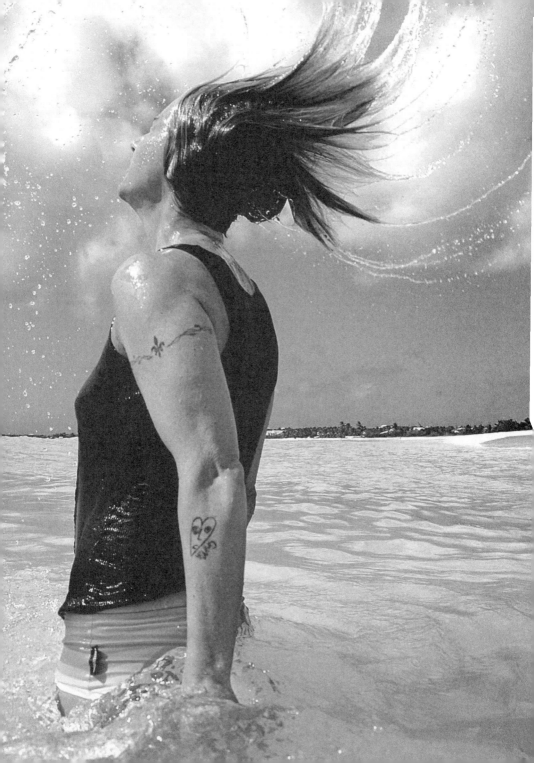

spiritual life, home life/physical environment, relationship with family/children, volunteer work. When you're ready and you're sitting there with the pencil, trying to decide where to put the X on your MAP, the first thing you need to do is ask yourself some important questions.

Start with what gives you a sense of fulfillment and joy versus what you feel is draining you. Look at each area of your life and figure out what is working for you and what isn't. What are you happy about and what are you unhappy about? Don't try to make a list on how to change things just yet—we will save that for later when we discuss goals—for now, just go with your gut instincts, your feelings in each of these areas.

Ask yourself this: Am I happy with my job? Am I happy in my life? Am I happy being single? Am I happy in my relationship? Am I happy with my dog? Am I happy with my children? Have I found my purpose? If the answer is no, then you have to ask yourself the even tougher question: Why not?

There can be many reasons why we aren't fulfilling our purpose or haven't figured it out yet. Sometimes it is because we are too practical and trying to do what we think we "should" be doing rather than what we want to be doing. Sometimes it is because we are afraid of pursuing our true purpose because we think we might fail. And sometimes we just need a little push in the form of emotional support. Acknowledge that you can't do it all on your own.

This is where the help comes in, because if you are not happy in your love relationship, you have to be able to ask

# PLAYLIST
## FOR FINDING YOUR PURPOSE

These songs are full of meaning about doing what you're meant to do.

| | |
|---|---|
| Alesso ft. Tove Lo | "Heroes" |
| Clean Bandit ft. Jess Glynn | "Rather Be" |
| Coldplay | "Fix You" |
| Justin Bieber | "Purpose" |
| Janet Jackson | "Special" |
| Parachute | "Something to Believe In" |
| Pharrell Williams | "Happy" |
| Rihanna | "We Found Love" |
| Snow Patrol | "Just Say Yes" |

your partner to give you some joy, or you have to ask them why they aren't acting happy to themselves and to you. (Which is probably why *you're* not happy, because we react to each other, right? It's all too easy for someone who's in a bad way to make you feel that way, too.)

Getting the help you need is the catalyst to you living a richer and fuller life. Inventory your spiritual practice today. What do you do to feel centered and grounded in the world around you? To me, that is at the root of what spirituality can be—nothing more complicated than your awareness and connection to the world around you and what's happening in it!

## LET FEAR FUEL YOU

The word *fear* is designed to put you on edge the minute you hear it, right? Well, being on edge can have its minuses, but it also has its pluses because it can spur you to action. So why not try embracing your fear instead of letting it hold you back? You can use it as a push.

Remember when you were at the swimming pool as a little kid, and your parents stood behind you and told you to jump? You were scared shitless, but they gave you a little nudge, knowing that you were going to be okay. While I got gently pushed, you may have been pulled, or maybe your parents let you stand there and cry and didn't make you go in if you didn't want to. However this kind of experience happened to you, we all had our first brush with fear, and this is where it all began. That gap between standing on the edge and landing in the water is pure fear. But now as an adult, you know you can jump right through it.

At least that's how I've learned to manage it. The way I've done so has been by talking about it. It took me decades to learn that avoiding discussing things, not sharing them, only makes the fear that much *worse.* You need to pick your go-to person and honestly discuss your situation with them, whatever it may be, and use them as a sounding board to strategize things. Talk about pros and cons, discuss potential outcomes, and share what you are afraid might or might not happen.

Usually, people get so into their own heads that they forget to share. Be vulnerable to people you trust. This totally helped me conquer my own fear. Maybe I see the fear a bit differently than you do. Once you jump through the fear, you're so happy, so empowered, so proud. Of course you can do it!

I learned all about pushing through fear thanks to Tony Robbins. He's got millions of fans for a good reason—he's a brilliant life coach. I met Tony through one of my Spinning students, Matthew, who was Tony's hairstylist. Mathew was a very chill rider, a very sanguine Brit, and as I watched him progress, his entire demeanor changed, along with his body. He went from barely being able to pedal to crushing the beat in true testimony. The class was definitely changing him.

After a ride one day, Matthew went to work with his adrenaline racing along with the endorphins, and he just happened to be cutting Tony's hair that afternoon. Tony, who is one of the most perceptive people on this planet, looked at him and said, "Whoa—what's going on?"

"Oh, nothing," Matthew replied.

"Really?" Tony went on "Who's the girl?"

Matthew laughed. "There's no girl. I promise you."

"*Something's* going on, because you've changed," Tony added. "Usually, people get really excited like you are right now because they're dating someone new."

"Well, maybe I'm in a sort of relationship with my Spinning instructor," Matthew said. "She reminds me a lot of you because she's so motivating and positive."

So Tony then kindly told Matthew to invite me to one of

his fire walks at his upcoming course. There was one coming up soon in Long Beach, California, for four days. With three thousand other people!

When Matthew told me this, I was thrilled. I started listening to Tony Robbins's color-coded cassette tapes in the 1990s. Like me, he'd come from nothing; he lived in a tiny apartment and did the dishes in his bathtub back in the days when he'd hand out fliers for his seminars. At first, he rented a little conference room and tried to get twenty people to show up and pay twenty bucks each to hear him speak. He started out with eight people and used the same approach I did. Start out with eight people, give them a guest pass, they come back and bring a friend next time for free. Then for Tony it went to forty bucks for forty people, then one hundred people, and then thousands. That's how he did it, and that's how I do it. Because "overnight success" is based on thirty years of hard work.

Tony's not hokey; he's cool and doesn't coddle you. He pumps your ass up. His course was like nothing I'd ever seen before. Tony was like a rock star; you'd have thought these people were going to see a Prince concert. The doors opened at the Long Beach Civic Auditorium, and because it was open seating, there were people literally sprinting to the front and climbing over seats to get close to the stage. Luckily, I was sitting in the VIP section in the front row with Matthew's sister (he'd already done the course) and Tony's family. It was one of the most energizing and motivating weekends of my life.

On day three, I think, came the fire walk across twelve feet of glowing-hot coals. If you stop, you burn; and if you push past the fear and just do it, you're fine. The trick is to chill your feet first so that your skin temperature drops, giving you an extra cushion of time before you might get burned. Once you take that first step, you keep moving. If you stop and look at the hot coals and freak out, you'll get burned.

It's amazing what your mind is capable of compelling your body to do. It's like watching little kids in a Tae Kwon Do class where four-year-olds can break a board with their tiny hands. You can do it when you know where to aim and how to follow through.

You can do it when you push past the fear.

After Tony's seminar and my fire walk, I realized I had to stop lying. I'd parked my tent in the liar's camp, as I called it back then, and I wanted to pack it up and go home to a healthier place. Like I said, when you are an addict, you do a lot of lying, starting with lying to yourself. So I went back to my apartment and told my then girlfriend that we had to fix things. I didn't want to do drugs anymore. I didn't want to drink anymore. And we did it. For nine months—until, like I told you, things went to shit the night before we left for Atlanta.

But I still know that if it weren't for Tony Robbins, I would not have been able to clear my emotional clutter. I would not be at SoulCycle. I would not be a sober, healthy person in a loving, giving relationship. I would not have a healthy body. I went to that seminar at the exact moment in my life when I needed someone to guide me so that I could push past the fears that were keeping me an addict.

## LEAVE YOUR COMFORT ZONE

Comfort is the killer of opportunity. The only way to get out of your comfort zone is by taking a risk.

Risk is one of those words, like fear, that makes most people click onto the negative, but I don't see it that way.

Risk-taking is throwing away the training wheels in your life while still taking a well-thought-out chance on yourself. Whatever it is you decide to do, you will see that visualizing yourself succeeding is one of the most empowering things you can do—I'll show you how in the next part of this book. Careful planning, complete execution, and follow-through on every level, as well as financial safety nets in place, trustworthy partners, and an intuition that this is the right decision, will be ingredients you will need to MAP it out. With those elements in place, you will be controlling as much of the risk as you can—and that makes the risk a lot less "risky."

"Stronger than you were yesterday, never as strong as tomorrow."

## IDENTIFY YOUR LUCK

Even when I was at my lowest point as an addict, I still felt lucky. Why? Maybe being on drugs does that to you, but for me, I knew it was a gateway for me to discover my true self. For me at least, part of what held me in the addiction was that I found my addicted squad. In my Los Angeles group, as you know already, we were all *functioning* addicts. Because everyone in our squad was doing the same thing, it was *sanctioned*; we all thought, and tried to convince ourselves, that it was okay. *At the time*. Looking back . . . maybe not so much.

It was only when I became a sober person that I realized my luck could have run out at any point during those years. Some of my friends died due to their drug habits. But here's the thing—even when you're enduring the very worst that can happen in life (loved ones dying, losing your job, needing to move, your children having problems, your partner wanting out, ill health), you can still feel lucky. You can still say to yourself, "I'm a good person, I'm going to make it, I'm going to figure myself out, I'm going to find my purpose." Realizing this can be incredibly empowering.

So I want you to think of the notion of luck not as an *external* notion, as in "Oh, he's so lucky because he was born rich" or "She's so lucky because she can eat whatever she wants and not gain any weight," but as an *internal* notion. A lot of people use the idea that they're not one of the lucky ones as an excuse to not push past fears or take risks. I don't agree with that. You make your own luck *inside*. You can choose to feel lucky.

Only you can identify your luck. The question you should ask yourself is, What do I feel lucky for? If you were standing at the gates of heaven, and had to tell Saint Peter what makes you lucky enough to pass through to paradise, what would your answer be?

Answering this question will also help you find your purpose, because you will be asking yourself what your most positive quality or talent is. Everyone has something special. You are lucky to have this. It's what makes you unique.

Even in my depths of despair after Michael's death, and my worsening addiction, yes, I was lucky. I was still alive. I'm not painting this picture like I was knocking on death's door by doing drugs—the thing people forget is that all it takes is one mishap, one drive home where you're not coherent, one wrong pill with the wrong pill with the wrong anything, and you're a goner. I wasn't in the despairing place Michael had been in, so deep and dark that he didn't want to live anymore. I feel lucky today to have had the strength to keep searching for the will to get me out of old patterns, even though it took me many attempts to do so. With the help of someone who really loved me, I did it.

Obviously, there will be bumps on your journey, but you're going to be like an Olympic gold medalist in freestyle skiing, navigating the moguls with finesse. I remember watching in awe the first time I ever saw that kind of skiing. *How do they*

*do it without falling and breaking their legs?* I wondere
realized it all had to do with purpose. Those skiers lo
they were doing. They trained their bodies to have the s
they needed. And most of all, they taught themselves how to
read the snow so they could find their way forward. They all
had the perfect combination of desire, physical strength, and
mental clarity. And you can, too.

---

SG TRUTH   **I use athletic metaphors in just about every single aspect of my life. I feel like it is one of the most relatable ways of
turning negatives into positives. You don't have to be an athlete to
do this, either!**

---

## MEDITATION FOR FINDING YOUR PURPOSE

This is a wonderful meditation when you feel the need for
guidance.

1. Sit in a comfortable room, in a cozy position, and take a few
   deep breaths. Close your eyes and raise your hands up toward the sky gently, with palms and heart open.
2. Ask the universe for some guidance here while your hands
   are up, and if you do this right now, I know—and the uni-

verse knows—you're serious about it. Open up to opportunity. Stay open to change; stay open to trust.

3. Concentrate on what you're asking for. You may have a very precise idea in your mind of what you want, or you may feel conflicted. It's important that you state to yourself what it is you want to happen. You can whisper it out loud. Keep your breathing steady.

4. Know deep in your heart that you'll get there. You'll get there because you're not going to stop until you do. There's no giving up anymore. Not only do you have a *can't stop, won't stop* attitude, you are not going to stop making and scoring goals for the rest of your life.

5. This is what ultimate vulnerability *is*. . . . Thinking like this is ultimate openness. This is you trusting whatever is out there that we don't understand. You cannot possibly comprehend all of it; there's too much. You have to rely on *that possibility that the space between what is and what isn't may have just what you need to get you where you need to go.* Have the faith that there is something bigger than you that is going to help you through and give you the help you need. Believe that there is something bigger than you that will protect you to make sure that you get through it. Trust me. It's there for you. For some it's God, Buddha, Jesus, Ganesh, Hanuman, or simply light. Whatever you do . . . believe in *something.*

6. Bring your arms back down and hold your hands together in your lap. Take a few more deep breaths.

7. Close the meditation out by seeing what you initially began with coming to fruition. See the entire scenario. See the smiles on the faces of everyone involved. The more you focus on this, the closer it will come to being your reality, especially if this is meant to be. Obviously, time, circumstances, and fate play a role here, but the key factor in these meditations is being honest about what you want the outcome to be. Let the universe take care of the rest. I truly believe that, because this meditation has worked for me on *many* occasions.

# PART II
# INTENTION

"Wake up . . .
show up . . .
live it up . . . !"

# THREE

## SETTING
## YOUR
## INTENTIONS

What does it mean to set your intentions? It means making a statement that represents your commitment to do something. I like to make these statements daily, or before any task, big or small, that helps me live in my purpose. It might sound simple, but this is an incredibly empowering process that clears your head so you can move forward. It forces you to slow down and focus on why you are doing what you are doing and how you are going to do it. It helps you to live life intentionally (get it?) instead of haphazardly. Knowing what your intentions are is the first step toward creating change in your life. Once you've made your intentions known, you can go about setting goals. I know that as someone with ADHD, if I don't do this, I'm screwed!

## STATE YOUR INTENTIONS

What do you need help with? What kind of power are you looking for? Do you have a tough issue at work you need to deal with? Are you trying to fit in your workout today? Are you about to sit in your car in traffic and all those bad drivers give you anxiety? Do you have a wedding to go to where you will have to deal with difficult family members?

Setting your intention gets you ready and psychs you up for the task at hand. It's saying, "Okay, I'm going to do this. I'm getting ready. I am focusing on the now." It's a little pep talk you give yourself about how you are going to handle a situation.

You set your intention by stating it out loud. Believe me, if you wake up in a grouchy mood and say, "I know I am going to have a bad day," you *will* have one. If, instead, you say, "I am not going to let this grouchy mood ruin my day. I am going to go for a run and then come back and eat a big bowl of blueberries with Greek yogurt and honey because that makes me feel good," you are going to undo the crappy mood and feel a whole lot better.

My goal with every class I teach is to encourage and empower my students to use their physical strength and fortitude to infuse every other aspect of their lives. In order to reach that goal, I *always* set and state my intentions before class starts. Either I set my intentions when I am taking the short walk from my apartment to the studio, or I shut the door to my office, and I turn off my phone because I need quiet and to be alone, without any interruptions. It's my time to focus and get my energy ready so I can power up. I'll close my eyes. Take a deep breath. Exhale, releasing anything I'm holding on to in my body, state my intention out loud ("I am going to give 100 percent of myself to make this a kick-ass class!"), and then I go right into choosing my music for that session.

Doing this for myself sets the tone for the class and for the rest of my students' day. I'm also choosing music that has a certain beat and feeling to it to reinforce the intentions I've decided upon. Some songs are so cheery you just want to sing along. Others are longer and slower, building up to an eventual crescendo subtly so that my students don't realize how hard they've been working to stay on the beat until the song is over.

For example, I once asked a friend who's a novelist how his process worked—where his plots and characters came from, what inspired him, how he did it. He told me that once he sorted out the general theme, he'd go to bed and start dreaming the characters, and then over time they would coalesce into more detailed scenes. He'd wake up and tell himself what he would write for the day. What he then added resonated with me the most: "I never actually put pen to paper until I know the general outline of the plot. Especially the ending. Some writers can write without a blueprint, but not me. I have to know where my characters are going in order to get them there."

What this writer was doing was creating a goal (to write a book). Without putting a name to what he was doing, he was setting his daily intentions to reach that goal. He went over his tasks in his head; he stated them aloud; he found his motivation; and he was then able to get to work.

Like this writer, start small with stating your intentions at first. All you need is a calm and quiet minute. What's most important it is to be alone and uninterrupted when you set up your intention for the day. It is you empowering yourself to get going.

Once you get used to setting intentions for a minute every morning you can increase the time you spend as you get more comfortable doing it. Your intention goal is fifteen minutes of meditation. You'll soon become so used to this kind of intense focusing that you will enjoy taking more time to do it. Eventually, this intention-setting time can be about visualizing yourself in these actual intentions—in other words, knowing what your intention is and picturing yourself living it.

When you set your intentions, not only will your work flow better, but you will be calmer and more focused when faced with the usual stresses of life. Instead of being anxious about your first meeting of the day (you know, the one with the unpleasant boss who always puts you on edge), your intention not to take this boss's comments personally will lesson your worries about your performance at work. Instead of dreading the commute home when you know you will be stuck in traffic, your intention to buy an audio book and listen to that instead will leave you calmer and less aggravated by the other drivers.

LYSU

In addition to stating your intentions aloud, I always say, "LYSU"—line your shit up! That means figuring out your tasks for the day. What are you doing after you leave for work? What is the most pressing issue you need to be prepared for? Do you have an important meeting? Is there an issue with your child's teacher? Is it an easy day when all you have to worry about is dusting the shelves in the living room, buying food for the dog, and having lunch with your boyfriend?

The Lineup Sheet is my version of a to-do list. Some Lineup Sheets will be easy, like a shopping list of tasks that take little energy or are fun to do. Some will be a little more complicated if you're dealing with matters that are sensitive. Line it up anyway, as this will help you keep your thoughts and your emotions in order and really assist with those I-am-overwhelmed sensations. Any time I have boxes to check, I turn it into a game, and I make sure I check all the boxes before the end of the day. Like this:

- DMV
- Call GMA
- Call Mom

For all your Lineup Sheets, get a piece of paper and a pen. You can't do this on a computer—you need to sit at a table and desk and focus on the paper.

---

**SG TRUTH** Since the dawning of the iPhone, I tend to do the boxes in my iPhone calendar, but it's not the same! Make the effort to write this down and make the boxes. It works! Post-its are great to fit in your wallet.

---

Here's what to do: On the right side of a piece of paper, write down what you have to do—call mom, call plumber, call little Johnny's teacher, send résumé to XYZ , go to FedEx, pay parking tickets, buy a book to read on vacation, send your friend who's sick some flowers.

Draw little squares to the left of each task. This way, when you check the box, you know you've put something in the pipeline of change. The more checked boxes, the happier you will be with your day.

What I'm doing here is trying to give you a bad-ass-y yet nice way to look at these lists. I know the word *task* is one of those clichéd kind of words and doesn't pack a lot of punch. So if, instead, we use the word *shit* with a positive attitude, and with a positive tone, it will put some velocity behind what you're doing. So say it with me: "I've got to line my shit up. LMSU!"

Feels good, right? You bet it does.

*What's the one thing I am never without? No, not a bottle of water. My favorite trusty little notebook. I'm always getting ideas, and I know that if I don't write them down, I may not remember them. Yes, I could use my phone, but when it comes to ideas, I prefer to write them rather than type them. Besides, having a notebook makes me more conscious of the fact that I am having ideas worthy of writing down—and that, in turn, spurs even more ideas.*

I LOVE MY NOTEBOOKS

Here's another scenario. Let's say you know you have to have an uncomfortable conversation with your spouse about things you want to do to liven up your relationship. Maybe your needs aren't being met anymore, and you're asking yourself, "Is it something *I'm* not doing in our relationship that's making my partner unhappy?"

You put on your Lineup Sheet: *What can we do to make our relationship awesome again?* When you line it up, think of things that you would be willing to do to make your partner happier. These could be to plan more things to do together, go out to dinner once a week, have more adventures, rub their feet when they get home after a long day, talk about more issues that are important to both of you, or have breakfast together every morning to fill each other in on daily events in your life, etc.

Coaches know all about LYSU; it's the whole point of training or rehearsing or studying. Someone throws the ball at you, you reach up to catch it, you slip, you fall, what are you going to do to recoup? You may fall nine times, but on the tenth time you are fearlessly up and running without hesitation. It's the long-term training requiring drills, practice, and repetition until you can easily catch the ball and run with it. Remember, everyone falls. Falling is *not failure*. Falling is part of the game of life.

As long as you have the instinct in your body to get up and try again, *you're going to be okay*. And you are going to realize that you are strong, and that no matter what happens in your life, *you're good*. That's the point of the Lineup Sheet. You have a plan, a list to hold you accountable for putting your life in motion. It is taking your intentions and giving yourself a list of things to do to help make them happen.

Stating your intentions and acknowledging the tasks required to fulfill them is what allows you to take the first turn of the knob toward a happier life. Your life revolves around *your* ultimate happiness and living with intention and taking the proper steps is how to tap into *your* happy, every single day.

---

SG TRUTH   Since I got my iPhone, I sometimes use Notes on it, but I always have a real notebook and a pen close by, too!

---

I think carrying the notebook is one of the best habits you can have. It will also help you take notes when you're reading this book, not just about my experiences, but about what I'm saying that particularly resonates with you in the moment you're reading it. You could write, for example, "Ideas of healing" or "Ask for help" or "Move it!" or "Get a jolt!" or anything that jumps out at you. You can keep these notes in the notebook or put them on Post-its and stick them where they're going to inspire you. Before you know it, you'll have entire notebooks full of amazing ideas that will inspire and motivate you, and you won't have to worry about accidentally erasing them the next time you hit the wrong key on your phone! And if your phone ever dies, you'll still have your notes!

## REINFORCING YOUR INTENTIONS WITH VISUALIZATION

Imagine that you have the power to visualize your destiny, and that today could be that day where you cross over into a new level of success in a more creative way, with out-of-the-box thinking and a unique approach to your goals. Imagine that for a second.

Time to visualize this success! In vivid, three-dimensional color, right down to the faded blue hue of your jeans and the soft and well-worn texture of your favorite T-shirt!

I would never be where I am today without visualization. I visualized myself as a teacher, as a loving partner, and as someone who kept quitting cigarettes until it eventually stuck. Of all the toxic things I gave up, smoking was by far one of the hardest. It took me five different times to visualize quitting, but I never gave up. A telling moment was when a seven-year-old found my cigarette butt in the toilet and shrieked through the house, "Someone was smoking!" So much for trying to hide that fail!

Let me be brutally open about this topic. It took me many, *many* failed attempts at quitting the toxic things I allowed into my life. (I have a method for quitting everything, but that is past the scope of this book—you can read about it in my next one!) This was due to me being what I called a triple-threat kinda gal. When I say that, I don't mean it in the athletic sense. I mean I had issues as a smoker, a drinker, and a drug user. It totally sucked. I hate admitting that, but the me now will never again be the me I used to be. There is not a chance in hell that I will go back to being Crazy Stacey ever again. Finally, after over ten years of being sober (with the help of my partner, my friends, my family, and my students), I am more connected to the sober version of myself than I was to the partying, crazy version of me.

Everything in your universe starts with what you think—your intentions—followed by your actions. You can *totally* push forward once you identify what you want. After you have stated your intentions, visualization allows you to see what you want in your mind's eye and turn it into reality. It clears your mind of all other thoughts except those you're focusing on with calm intent. This lets your brain do the work for you. During visualizations, you can watch a movie in your mind based on all your new ideas of what you want in your life.

Your visualization can be an image of something positive

("I want a new job") or something you are trying to overcome ("I want to stop smoking"), or anything at all. It's like Mad Libs, that fill-in-the-blank game you probably played when you were younger. What I'm going to show you how to do is play out the scenario in your head, imagining yourself in that situation attaining the results you seek. I want you to visualize every step of the way, down to the color of the shoes you are wearing and the jewelry on your wrist during the handshake you make with your boss when he promotes you and gives you a raise, to the ecstatic blush on your cheeks and the jubilant e-mail you send to your friends with the good news.

When you are finished with your visualization, bring your attention back to your breathing and slowly begin to come back to your body and the space you are in. Sit up tall. Your breathing might have changed, along with your body position. You might feel energized, or you might be a bit tired. These are all normal responses, and show you how powerful the visualization actually was.

Remember your feelings of confidence, success, and achievement. Remember how vivid the images were and how mentally tough and inspired you feel. And because you wrote the script, you can recall these images and feelings anytime you choose.

Look, it's totally normal that doing visualizations may feel weird in the beginning. It takes a pretty grounded, centered, and ready person to sit and visualize. I understand if you aren't ready, and I also understand if you're not into them. No big-are here for those of you who need calm in your life, help focusing and manifesting some things. I'm not expecting my friend Deepak to read this and go, "Oh, I never thought of that." These practices have been used for thousands of years—I'm just packaging them my way!

If you have trouble with visualizations at first, don't worry. It's a learned skill, and like any other skill, it can sometimes take a while for you to learn. One way is to try picturing your favorite photo—of *you*. I believe in motivational fridge pics if they are of you in a happy place, not a retouched photo of a supermodel or a fitness guru.

## Visualization for Empowerment

This is a very grounding visualization that will empower you by setting a positive vibration for your day.

1. Close your eyes and sit in a comfortable position, in a spot where you won't be interrupted. Imagine you are at the beach on a glorious summer's day. Can you feel the soft breeze and taste the tang of the salty sea air? Of course you can!
2. Take your surfboard (yes, you—even if you don't know how to swim or are scared of the big waves, you can imagine yourself out there in the surf) and run into the sea. Picture yourself lying flat on your tummy, easily paddling out past the shore break, the first set of waves. Turn yourself around now and face the shoreline, powerfully waiting for the next set.
3. Wait for the ideal wave, then pop up on your feet. You're in

charge. You're balanced perfectly on the board, without a hint of fear. You soften your stance a little bit, confident of your position.

4. You ride the wave all the way back to the shore. It feels like you're flying. You've never felt so alive, with the sound of the ocean and the splash of water on your feet, and your body so utterly in tune with the board and the wave beneath you.

5. You arrive safely back on the beach, exhilarated and proud of your strength.

6. And then you go out there and do it again.

Feels pretty good, doesn't it? You can do this visualization in just a minute. You can even ride a longer wave for as long as you need to. Or, if you want, you can switch it up and insert mountain climbing, white-water rafting, or downhill skiing into your visualization. Just find something that you can easily picture—maybe something on your bucket list, like a hot-air balloon ride or skydiving—that brings powerful imagery into your head. I want you to be happy in the visualizations. This is never supposed to feel like a chore. It's a vibration tool, and it helps you focus on power.

Remember, this is a chosen visualization to change the vibration of your body. If you visualize yourself strong in the ocean, or on a mountain, or anywhere there is powerful movement, your inner vibration could possibly change the way you move in your actual reality. Don't judge it, just try it. You may be surprised at how well visualizations *work*!

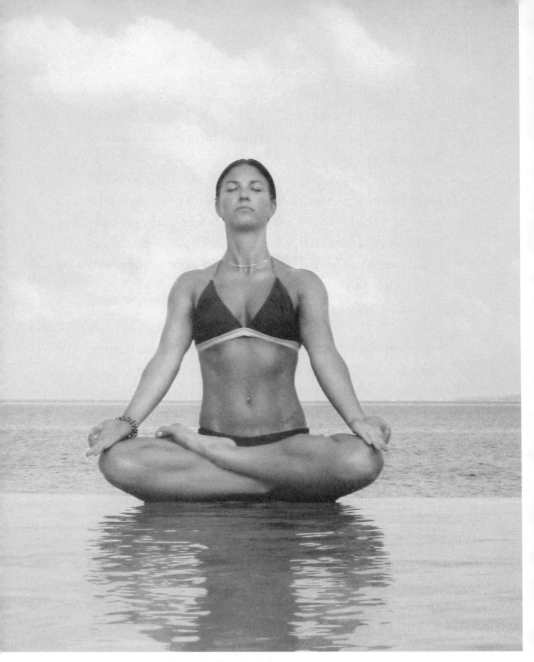

In the Maldives (Islands), 2001

Visualizations are there to empower you. If you find it's too hard or too boring to do without music, go for it. Play your favorite song or songs when you're doing your visualizations and meditations. There's no reason they don't deserve a soundtrack!

## Visualization for Creativity and Focus

Do this visualization before you start work on the days you feel you need it. The goal is to find a healthy and consistent routine.

---

**SG TRUTH** I have to confess, I have gotten out of practice with my own visualization time. I used to do it every day, when I had far fewer responsibilities and a less fraught schedule. Now I do this maybe once or twice a week in my office when I'm alone. I need to work a lot harder on doing this every day!

---

1. Close your eyes. You are going to see yourself performing at a high level of creativity and focus and drive. You are centered and balanced. No matter what you've done in the past, it won't matter today, because today is a brand-new version of you. Today you have more power, more influence, more integrity. You're in the positive zone. Stay there.
2. Think about something that you really want in your life. Something that you're going for. Something you're trying to achieve. Something you're trying to finish. Something

you're trying to start. Think about something like that. Something that inspires you, gets you excited, gets you motivated. Something good. You got it? Is it there? Do you see it? *Do it now.*

3. Picture you embracing what it is you want. Find that wonderful space between being scared and not being scared. That place is called *trust*.

4. If you struggle with finding that space, focus on your breath. The most consistent thing you can ever do is breathe, and it is an action that you can control in nearly all circumstances. It will get you through *everything*.

## Visualization for Energy and/or Love

This is a terrific visualization to do before a class of any kind, before a meeting at work or school, or in any group situation.

1. Close your eyes and relax your forehead, your cheeks, your lips, your neck, your arms, your fingers. Then focus on your breath for a few seconds. As you breathe, feel your forehead relax, your eyebrows, your eyelashes, your cheeks, your lips. Let your tongue sit in the bottom of your mouth, softly, away from pushing up against your teeth. Relax your neck. Relax your shoulders. Sit up tall. I want you to be so grateful, grateful for your life, your health, your wellness; the very blessing that brought you to this moment is the one that will fuel you for the entire day. *Do this now.*

2. Imagine you are with a like-minded, supportive group of

people. There is, as you know, a tremendous power in a group collective. We are all energies, after all. We are all force fields walking through this universe. And when you capture this many amazing attitudes, it's like that magic moment when your children are collecting fireflies, running around while shouting with giggles, joyfully watching the lights flicker on and off in the darkness in the jar full of life and love.

3. Keep your eyes closed and imagine your special jar of life and love. As you feel it in your heart, let it heal you. And then you have the light of love to heal everybody you touch. This is how we change the world, and this is how we move toward our intentions and our goals.

4. Feel your body glow, getting brighter and brighter. Brighter and brighter. One more deep breath here for transformation. *Do this now.*

5. Open your eyes. You are now flooded with energy, ready to tackle any situation.

## MOVING MEDITATIONS

When I studied yoga in India, it was difficult for me to master a lot of the moves at first, in large part because I am the kind of person who is in perpetual motion. Once I figured out that if I combined the calming wonderfulness of yoga/meditation techniques with *movement,* I had the best of both—for *me*. That's what I transformed into my teaching methods, and it's a large reason my classes are so successful. My students are moving as hard as they possibly can, but they learn how to calm their minds even when their hearts are pumping and the sweat is blurring their eyes.

Say "meditation" to someone, and they usually picture someone sitting in a quiet, dark room. But you can just as easily meditate, relaxing yourself and visualizing, while your body is in motion during a Moving Meditation. It's where the real you pops out. It's when your true integrity, drive, passion, perseverance, tenacity, grace, and patience start to show and shine.

When you do any tasks—emotional, as in dealing with a loved one; or physical, such as a workout—with all the positive affirmations of the Moving Meditations, it's almost a perfect storm. It's like a satisfying stretch for your brain, which is hearing the affirmations while you're feeling and pushing through a physical hurdle or boundary or challenge. Add the rhythm of music to the mix, and you're transported to an almost trancelike state while in motion.

I created these Moving Meditations after I had been teaching for a few years, and they work wonders for centering and balancing who you are on a cellular level, as a human being. Once you master Moving Meditations, whether you're walking, running, jogging, swimming, biking, or doing any kind of exercise, you'll come back to them day after day after day. Not only do they make you feel (and look) better, but they're really *fun*!

These can be done during any kind of workout where you

Our driver, Shisa, Mysore, India

will be safely in motion—in an indoor cycling class, on a re-cumbent bicycle, on a treadmill or rowing machine, or while walking on level ground. What you're reading now is exactly how I talk to my students when they're riding in class. Imagine that it's my voice speaking to you. Or go ahead and read these aloud into a voice recorder, and play them as you move.

Obviously, you can't meditate and read this book at the same time. If you want help with decision-making, I suggest you read through these meditations once or twice, and then give them a shot. If some of the words written here really strike you, I encourage you to let that process flow and dive in.

## Moving Meditation for Setting Your Intentions

1. Picture yourself in a meadow with the green grass soft un-der your feet and the sky a stunning blue. The sun is bright but not blazing, making you feel all aglow as you turn your head up toward it.
2. Imagine one large, white, puffy cloud floating up in that blue, blue sky. That's it. Your meditation. When you start to feel a thought come through your mind, I want you to put it on the cloud and watch it gently float away.
3. After it's gone, put another fresh cloud right there. This is how you reset your mind. You are pushing away the old thoughts and replacing them with new, loving, and amazing thoughts.

4. Next, you are at the beach, walking strong on the firm white sand in the body you've always wanted for yourself.

5. You've never felt more confident in your intentions as you transform back to yourself, striding in and out of the water and walking on the sand again.

6. Time is barely moving, but you're strong enough to get through it now. You're strong enough to push through—it's who you are. Strong, determined, tenacious, focused, reliable, consistent, honest, truthful, and beautiful. You keep moving until you reach the house at the end of the beach, the welcoming house that you realize is your home, and when you put your hand on the doorknob, take a deep breath and come back to reality.

## Moving Meditation to Help with Decision-Making

1. Before you start, make sure you're thinking positively. Make sure you are in it to win it with your thought process. Get into a zone with yourself, and focus on your breath. This is not about anybody else but you. This is your time. Close your eyes and feel your own power—the very power you were born with.

2. Open your eyes, take a few deep breaths, and *relax*. Before anything will make sense you have to find your center of gravity. So relax your shoulders. Drop your head and relax

...orehead, relax your eyebrows, relax your cheeks, relax your neck, relax your biceps, relax your chest.

3. Say this mantra silently: *Can't stop, won't stop trying, can't stop, won't stop pushing, can't stop, won't stop movin' and groovin' and workin' and pushin'.* (Today! Remember you can't meditate for tomorrow today. You have to take each day on its own.) Play *those* words in your head over and over and over. It will help you find some pep in your step, and rush your adrenaline a little bit to give you the motivation you need for whatever reason you went on that walk in the first place.

4. Now let's put a visual in front of your head. Keep your pace with however you're moving. Don't slow down. *Can't stop, won't stop trying, can't stop, won't stop pushing, can't stop, won't stop movin' and groovin' and workin' and pushin'.* There's got to be somewhere that you go in your head when you want peace . . . and on that stretch of road where you go for peace, I want you to keep yourself right there, keep the pace, and see what it is you really want for yourself.

5. Visualize holding on to yourself—hug yourself from the inside out. Sometimes there's no one around to give you a hug when you need it, so you hug yourself by flexing your abs really tight. This just involves tightening your abs and hugging yourself almost like you're bracing for someone to hit your tummy. That's a self-hug! *Can't stop, won't stop trying, can't stop, won't stop pushing, can't stop, won't stop movin' and groovin' and workin' and pushin'.*

6. Be careful what you're thinking about here. You have a lot

of power right now with this mental behavior. It's a direct shot into the universe when you have this much going on. I can almost guarantee if you have a positive thought going on and don't stop thinking that powerful thought and push through, there will be something magical, such as a long-awaited message in your voicemail, waiting for you when the Moving Meditation is over. Stay 100 percent prime-time in love with the thought. Don't let anything else penetrate, or it won't work. If you stay focused on it and punch it through, it will work.

7. Keep your breathing even and keep playing the mantra in your head until you feel it's a great time to stop.

## Moving Meditation to Help You Work Out and/or for Emotional Strength

1. Every time you choose to move, it's your choice where you're going to take yourself. Every day is a different twenty-four hours. There's a different vibration on every hour of every day, so you have to lock in to your highest vibration here and now. Don't forget that *you* are the vibration.

2. Self-mantra: Say to yourself, *This is my life. I own it. It belongs to me. I am going to live it the way I want to. I am going to make it an awesome day. My body is strong and it is mine and I am going to use it to make me stronger.*

3. Feel the strength flood your body from your head down to your toes. It's an attitude, it's a motivated approach for your

life. It's emotion, it's activity, it's energy, it's electricity, it's vibration, it's who you are. Walk, run, ride a bike, jump up and down in your kitchen, just *move*. And keep on moving. Sometimes a fist in the air and a nice loud "YEAH!" can do the trick!

4. You were born with a voice—make sure you use it at least once a day. Communication is key. How you deliver your words is crucial. You can't go wrong if you're delivering those words from a perspective of strength and kindness.

5. It's your choice. If there's something you're really going for in your life, I want you to put it out there and believe it will happen. This is where your true colors start to shine through. Your true testimony to yourself, what you really believe in, how you handle all the challenges in your life is going to show right here from wherever you are, whether it's up or down. You're pushing through this day. What will you choose to do today? Make it a productive one!

6. If there were no boundaries, if there were no consequences, if there were no limitations, where would you go now? Change your attitude now. Shift it to higher levels of thinking, a stronger belief system, with more integrity, more honesty. Be the best you in this imagery. Remember, your cells are listening to what your mind says. The more positive you are with your thoughts, the better your body feels.

7. Stay focused, stay driven, stay in your Moving Meditation until you feel it's a great time to stop.

Now is a good time to make a fist and punch the air and yell in a whisper that is strong and meaningful, "YEAH!"

## ASK THE UNIVERSE FOR HELP

Stating your intentions works. The thing is, not enough people *really* do it because it takes a bit of work—and to be *on it,* it takes a small bit of nonjudgmental belief that there are forces in the universe willing to help you if you ask for it.

I am going to walk you through a Moving Meditation where you ask the universe for help in landing the job you not only want but need very badly. You can then tweak this scenario for any other goal in your life. Believe in this technique whole-heartedly and it *will* work for you.

All you need is a piece of paper, a pen, and a small white candle.

1. On the piece of paper, write down your goal—in this case, it's "I Am Going to Get a Fabulous Job at XYZ." (Write in very small print because you're going to fold the paper up.) Under the main goal, write down everything positive you can think of about this job, even if you know that position may not exist *yet*. Here are some examples for you to choose from: "I will love this job. This job will be close to where I live. My boss will be incredible. My salary will be what I de-

serve. I am worthy of getting this job. I am going to find this job. This job is right for me. Somebody needs me to do this job. I am the right person for this job." (Notice how your thinking will shift from "I need a job" to "I am the right person for this job" to "I'm going to get this job." Your mental determination is already shifting!)

2. Fold the paper in half and put it underneath the white candle. (Be sure, of course, that it's sitting flat and won't tip!) Light the candle, and as you sit by it and stare into the flame, go through all the items on your list and try to remember as many of them as possible. Say them out loud.

3. Get up, make your wish that the universe hears your intention (in this case, for the job), blow out the candle, and go walk around the block. This is *very* important. Even if it's just to the end of the street and back—even in the rain or snow—you must get outside and *move* so the universe knows that you're putting your intentions into action. In other words, the instant you uptake this list, it's there in your mind, and you want to telepathically tell the universe that you're serious. Again . . . you gotta believe or this will absolutely *not* help you.

Call me cuckoo for Cocoa Puffs all you want, but this shit works. I have many, many testimonials to prove it. Seriously! Have faith. *Believe*. It will happen.

4. You are going to repeat step 3 every freaking day until that job shows up. You don't stop. (Okay, so if there's a blizzard or hurricane outside, or if you're not feeling well, open your

door, go through your intention list, and then close it and go back inside—no other excuses allowed!) It might take one day, it might take a week, it might take a month, or even a year or two years—but you don't stop until that job shows up.

"Don't scoff at asking the universe for help."

## Get Ready to Shine and Pop

While you're putting your energy and desire for this job out into the universe, you are also going to work on your visualization in preparation for the day when the fateful phone call or e-mail arrives telling you you've got an interview. Follow these steps. They're really good training for any kind of important meeting.

1. In your mind, go through your closet. What are you going to wear to your appointment or interview? Make sure when you visualize yourself, you look great. Don't hesitate to put yourself in an outfit you don't even own—it could be something you saw in a store window or in a magazine that you wish you could have. Whatever it is, just make sure that you feel good in it.

2. Then when you visualize what you're wearing, visualize how you're getting to where you're going. If you have an interview a mile away or an interview in a specific office building or someone's house, imagine yourself getting there with absolutely no traffic. All the lights are green. It's a beauti-

ful day outside in your visualization, even if it's raining or snowing right now. Just clear a path and think, *Green lights, green lights*. When you arrive at your visualized destination, there is a parking spot right in front with your name on it. The parking gods are on your side, and you don't even have to think about parallel parking!

3. Next comes what I think is one of the most important visualizations, one I always do: Imagine the person you're supposed to meet is smiling as they greet you. They're smiling with pleasure as they shake your hand and show you to your seat. They are so happy to see you. You instantly feel confident and enthusiastic.

4. As soon as you sit down, imagine that the conversation is going totally in your favor. They tell you yes, they would love to have you at this job, what great ideas you have, they love what you bring to the table. This is going to be amazing for the entire staff. Then they thank you, shake your hand again, and say good-bye with a proud and contented smile for the brilliant choice they have made—namely, hiring *you*.

When you set that deep of an intention—with anything that you're about to do—it really gives it the opportunity to line up. It tells the universe that this is what you want, and it creates an unknown path. Since we as humans don't really know how our telepathic powers manifest, why not just tell the universe how it's supposed to go down? Because then at least you have set the path in motion. The way you tune in to this energy is by repeating your visualizations over and over. You will literally be creating your own destiny. And instead of saying, "I want this job later or soon or next month," you will always be saying, "I want this job now, immediately." Be positive. Be confident. After all, if you don't ask, how can you get what you want?

Please don't scoff at asking the universe for help. If you do, it's like a double negative. Because not only are you *not* asking, but you're stripping your request of its power. Picture a magnet that is attracting all your intentions when you are thinking positive and visualizing, and then the second you don't believe, the magnet reverses its charge and everything is instantly repelled.

You shine when you try. You shine when you pay attention. In other words, you pop! You want to live that way—shining and popping! That's why making your list, writing down your goals, and setting your intentions is so important to do by hand, on paper. To say it out loud and to put it in motion. Ask yourself: If there were no boundaries, no consequences, and no limitations, where would you go now?

After all, as Roald Dahl wrote in his book *The Minpins,* "Those who don't believe in magic will never find it."

"A week
is seven
brand-new
days to
be stronger."

# FOUR
## DEFINING
## YOUR GOALS

Once you have learned to set intentions, you are ready to take the next step toward realizing your goals. In this chapter, I'll show you how to identify and define your personal and professional goals. Then, I'll explain how to reinforce them with powerful fine-tuning techniques.

How do you define your own goals? What do you want to achieve? There are many ways to begin. If you need inspiration, you can use your five senses so that your goals are revealed in a way that works for you. If one of your senses is stronger than the others, you might want to start with that approach, or you can use all the approaches in whatever order you like. I

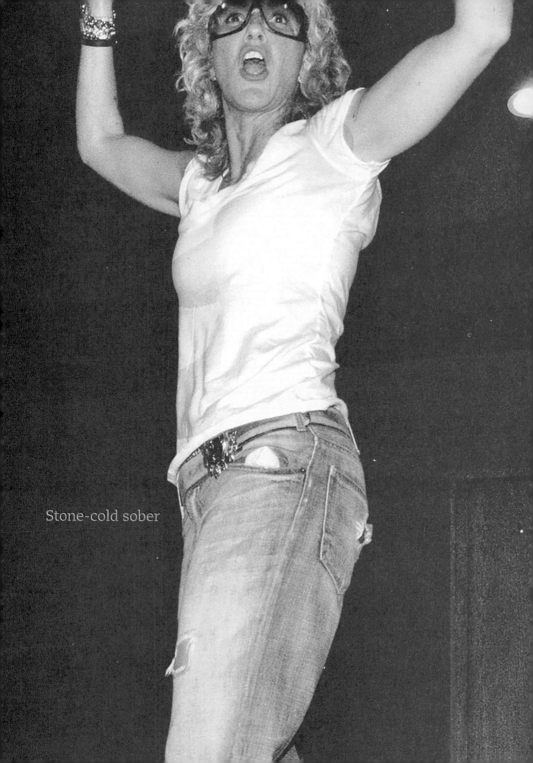

Stone-cold sober

find that they all work for me, and at different times, different methods work better than others.

What I mean when I say this is that some of us do better when we use lists, some of us love to make vision boards, some of us like to go to sessions with a therapist, some of us have coffee with a mentor, some of us talk to our parents about things, some of us go for a long walk . . . whatever it is that gets you in that *zone* of who you really are . . . that's the zone I need you to get into when you start thinking about what your real goals are and how to reach them.

## USING YOUR FIVE SENSES TO DEFINE AND REINFORCE YOUR GOALS

---

**SG TRUTH** My entire office is one big vision board. Some people love to make a specific one and hang it on a wall; I curate mine on my desk with live inspiration items, books, little figurines of people I love, quote cards, magazines I've written in, etc.

---

## SIGHT: Make a Vision Board

A useful way to visualize your goals is with a vision board.

Clothing designers create incredible vision boards for their new collections every season. Betsey Johnson, for example, puts up swatches of fabrics and trims, different colors and textures, all kinds of sketches, photographs, and drawings of things that inspire her. Screenwriters take index cards with all the scenes in their movies, put them up on a board, and move them around until the flow of the story is correct.

What a vision board does is allow you to see your goal manifested and on display in front of you at all times so you have constant reinforcement for your goals. You can make yours out of any materials—just pick a medium that feels good in your hand. I know a lot of people who use chalk and a board/wall that's been covered with chalk paint so they can easily update their ideas. But you don't have to go that big if you don't want it. Your vision board can be the size of an envelope if you want it to be.

Get creative with your vision board. Place your goal at the top, and surround it with images and/or words that inspire you. Write down your daily or weekly mantra and pin it up. Look for enticing photos or drawings that make you feel good or represent your goals. Be sure to do it by hand, as this will help you focus. The only tool you really need is whatever you're writing with, some magazines, and some tape or glue.

Remember, you can modify this idea to suit your style. There are no rules, except to do whatever you like and have fun. When you reach your goal, keep the vision board as a memento, if you like, and start a new one. And remember, you can curate a vision section on your desk as well, which is what I do. I wanted to give you options here so you realize how easy it is.

## TOUCH: Make a Meditation Station

A Meditation Station is a small place where you can sit and meditate and do your visualizations undisturbed. Your Meditation Station can be on your desk at work, at home, or both.

I have a special table in my office that belonged to my beloved grandma Mary Lou that has my Meditation Talismans on it. These are objects that are incredibly special to me and charged with meaning. I use them to help me set my intentions, nourish my spirit, and focus on my goals. They include a rosary and a small statue of a saint I got at the mission in Carmel, California, when I rode my bike from San Francisco to Los Angeles and we had to stop there; sandalwood beads from India from one of my students; sandalwood protection oil; the Hindu gods I got with Kelly of Ganesh and Hanuman; the Hindu goddess Lakshmi; a tiny statue of Buddha; a crystal from Ellen; my eight-year sobriety chip from Weezie; and a round silver plate that was my grandma's that says *love, love, love* all around the outside of it. This table is literally covered with love!

Your own talisman should be a goal-defining object that is important to you, one that you will associate with power and perseverance. It can be a crystal or a rosary or Tibetan prayer beads, as many people find the repetitive motion of running the beads through their fingers to be instantly soothing and stress-relieving—it's sort of like listening to music but with your fingers. It can be something you found on a family vacation, or a family heirloom like a cuff link from your grandfather. I like to use a small rock I found on a beach. Whatever you choose is going to have a vibration that's going to resonate with you. It's deeply personal and never needs to be explained to anybody. Think of it as your lucky charm.

If you don't have the space for a table or want to keep it private, place your talismans in a soft little bag in your purse or a drawer and pull them out when you need to. You can also find or buy talismans in multiples and keep them in your desk drawer, your backpack, your gym bag, your car, and at home.

---

**SG TRUTH** I have them everywhere for protection. I never travel without my pocket edition *Zohar* from the Kabbalah Centre here in New York, and I always have some type of Hindu god tucked in a pocket of my luggage.

---

Since I started using my Meditation Station, my brain has been less scattered and I find it much easier to focus. My message to my students and the community seems more grounded every day. I know this is going to happen for you, too.

## TASTE: Meditation Station Tea

How can you use your sense of taste to define your goals?

Simple—with a special Meditation Station tea. The purpose of this drink is to reinforce your mind-set and determination to reach your goals. After a very short while, you will begin to associate the taste of this drink with setting your intentions. Sip an energizing tea before a workout or when you're doing any Moving Meditation, if possible; choose a calming tea when you're visualizing at your Meditation Table. Teavana Oprah Decaf Chai and DavidsTea are awesome, and you can order them and many other varieties online.

Getting into the tea habit is a win-win, as you'll not only get the hydration you need and something to fill you up without any calories, but the therapeutic value of whatever is in the tea. Your Meditation Station tea should be caffeine-free. Try to drink it without any sweetener, so find a flavor you really like. I like my Oprah Chai hot, but you can make it the night before and refrigerate it if you prefer iced tea.

And for those of you who really don't like tea, use cold or hot water with lemon instead.

## SMELL: Spiritual Bath

Nothing is more potent than the power of scent. It's the only one of our senses that is hardwired to go right to our brain. No wonder the waft of a certain perfume can instantly transport you back to your mother's bedroom as you sat watching her get ready for a night out, or take you back to the first time you made confetti cake or kissed someone in high school. For me, it's Red Vines, the kind of chewy candy you get at the movies. One whiff and I'm instantly transported back to 1977, where I'm sitting in the front row of the theater with Scott Martinez and Robby Starnes, when the now famous theme to *Star Wars*

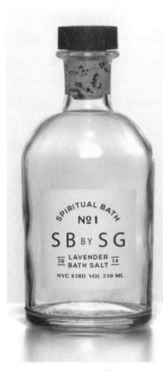

Spiritual Bath by
Stacey Griffith

begins, and I am off to another galaxy.

Warm water recalibrates your vibration, especially when it's scented. Use your time in the bath not just for stress relief, but to help you focus on your visualizations. The beauty of the bath is that we, as humans, all started in water. That's why it's so soothing and so empowering.

Scent is so important to me that I created my own Spiritual Bath products. My mom was a big bath taker, so I grew up loving a long soak. As I got older, I started creating a bathroom environment with scented bath salts and candles, and I got the name for my products when my partner's children asked me to make them because my baths always smelled so good. They'd get in the warm water and I'd light all the candles and they'd go, "Oh, it's so spiritual in here," and I'd smile and say, "It's spiritual bath time!" Their friends would come over, put their bathing suits on, and dash into the bathroom. I'd light a whole bunch of candles and a stick of incense, and then say, "Okay, the rule of the spiritual

Something I'd like you to think about is the difference between
*spirit* and *spiritual*. Especially as these words are often misused
ing true beliefs, perhaps, to someone who's merely having a tre
a spa.

*Spirit* is defined as the soul, or character or ethos. A spirit can also be a
ghost; spirits are alcoholic; *spirited* means full of energy or secretly con-
veyed away. *Spiritual* is defined as being related to the spirit or soul, or a religious belief. It's synonymous with enlightenment—or at least it should be.

The point is, don't get freaked out if you aren't "spiritual" in the religious
sense. Spirituality has many meanings and definitions. I would say it's far
more important to be connected to a higher level of consciousness than
anything else, in touch with a deeper level of yourself—a cellular level, if
you will. That's what will bring connectedness. The more connected you
are to your core beliefs as a person, the more balanced and loving your
vibration will be.

bath is that you have to whisper in here, and you can only talk
about things that make you happy." Then I'd hand them one
sweet treat, like a small piece of candy, and leave them to their
blissful soak.

The first kit I made for adults was for Oprah, as a thank-you
after the "Life You Want" tour in 2014, because I knew she loves
her baths as much as I love mine. It was like creating a Meditation Station with bath salts, a scrub, a foaming bath ball,
incense, Epsom salts, washcloths from Brunello Cucinelli in

Italy because I knew she adored them, eight votive candles that represented the eight letters in "I love you," and very expensive caramels as the sweet treat. In my note, I told her to eat only one caramel per bath, to light the votives safely, and to light the incense, make a wish, then blow it out.

I gave it to her at the wrap party the last night we were together, and she left me a voice mail that I have saved to this day. She told me how much she loved and appreciated this gift, and thanked me as only she could for sending it to her. (I have to add, I was *dying* after hearing this—who gets messages from Oprah on their voice mail?!)

The products I chose to create in my SB by SG line are fresh-scented bath gels like citrus for daytime and jasmine for nighttime; Epsom salts for soaking those sore muscles; and eucalyptus and lilac bath salts.

Have fun creating your own scented environment—in the bath, and wherever you like. Choose a signature scent, inhale deeply, and enjoy the moment. Then focus on your intentions.

## HEARING: Music Is the Soundtrack to Your Life

I have more than 32,000 songs on my computer. They're all part of my playlist. Music is an integral part of my life, every day, and it should be an integral part of yours, too.

Before I started working as a trainer, I had a lot of DJ friends in Los Angeles. For my thirty-third birthday, they all pitched in and bought me turntables and showed me the basics. I turned my spare bedroom into a studio and taught myself how to DJ, and then enrolled at the Music Institute in Hollywood, California, to become a sound engineer. I loved music so much and wanted to learn how to record and remix. I thought that kind of work would been an ideal career for all my skills.

Unfortunately, I was so messed up on drugs that I couldn't finish school, especially when I got gigs where someone would ask me fly to Miami and DJ a party on the day of an exam. Despite this, my DJ training has always helped me structure my classes. The more music you have—and the louder you can play it (unless your neighbors and your ENT doc complain)—the better!

I don't think anything is a better motivator for any task or goal than harnessing the power of music. It gets you *moving*. During a workout, it helps you push harder, it jacks you up to the next level, and then it relaxes you while you wind down. It helps you head toward that zone where you are totally inside the song, perfectly in sync with your body. When my class gets quiet, I know my students are really feeling the music. I always tell them to put their bodies *inside* the music, and then stay on top of the rhythm while we're pedaling to the beat. Let the music do the job, and ride it like a wave.

During any other time, music can be used to set, enhance, or change a mood, bringing your energy level down (*not* on my recommended list!) or soaring up higher than you ever thought possible. Music transports us. One study found college students who exercised to music experienced an increase in creative fluency—they were better able to generate different types of ideas. (And their butts looked great, too!) If you've had a really shitty time at work and all you want to do is get in your car with a new download, shut your phone off, crank up the volume, and drive away, it's because you know you're going to be safe in your little cocoon, sloughing off the stresses of the day.

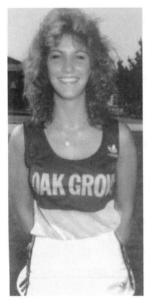

High school cross country

### Identify Your Theme Song

When I was in high school, I ran varsity cross country for the school team. Walkmans hadn't come out yet so I had to sing a song in my head that was perfect timing for my feet. The one that always worked for me was Fleetwood Mac's "Tusk," and the line I sang over and over and over again was, "Don't tell me that you love me . . ." because it had an awesome beat to it. I'd sing those lyrics, and when I got tired I'd pretend there was an imaginary rope I could grab on to that would pull me up the hill—I was visualizing without even realizing what I was doing! Even now, whenever I hear that song I am instantly transported back to San Jose, California, up in those mountains on those dirt trails, singin' that song in my head, over and over.

# PLAYLIST

## MY FAVORITE PUMP-YOU-UP-TO-GET-MOTIVATED SONGS

These are some of my favorite songs that get me going . . . and going . . . farther than I thought possible, with a reflection at the end, ha-ha! (That's for my over-forty crew!)

| | |
|---|---|
| Christopher Cross | "Never Be the Same" |
| Earth Wind & Fire | "September" (James Egbert Remix) |
| Eos, Steve Aoko, Chris Lake, David Guetta | "Play Boneless Hard Alive" |
| Jess Glynn | "Rather Be" |
| Ariana Grande | "Be Alright" |
| Demi Lovato | "Confident" |
| Madonna | "Burnin' Up" |
| Nom De Strip vs. Breach | "Techno Jack" |
| Christina Perri (remix album) | "Human" |

"Tusk" became my theme song at the time, when I really needed one. Moviemakers know how important they are, too. That's why *Rocky* and *Star Wars* have such iconic theme songs, to represent the energy and the vibration of the movie. Of all the different scenes in a film, it only takes a few minutes of one song to represent them.

Your own theme song can be whatever you like, and it can

change over time, too. It can be the song that gets you going in the morning, the song you love to put your makeup on to. It can be the song that's the trigger to get you moving for your workout or when you're cleaning the house or sitting down to pay the bills. It's the song you set as your ring tone, so that every time somebody calls you, you're reinforcing your theme. (And it will also help you pick up the phone!)

Whenever you need a pep talk for conquering whatever intentions or goals you have set, put on your theme song. It's there to give you courage. If you're going on a job interview or a date or prepping for a meeting that is making you anxious, play it several times. You already know it's the song that works, that represents your best you. Then go for it.

And don't forget to play your theme song at the end of every workout, as a celebration cue that you did all the work you said you were going to do. Well done!

### Make Your Own Mixtapes . . . Yes, I Said Mixtapes!

Even if I'm in the worst possible mood, I never play sad breakup or emo songs, because they bring me down. I can snap myself out of a state because I make sure to play music that has a happy, sexy, beachy kind of vibe that reminds me of sunshine. It makes me feel good.

You can easily do the same thanks to digital technology. Simply make your own mixtapes to help you set your intentions and get you moving. You can tailor the beat of your songs: a faster one for energy and then a slower one to chill out. Music to distract you from your afternoon sugar cravings; music to give you courage. It is quite amazing how you can begin to amp up the challenge in your workouts just by picking faster-tempo songs. Try googling songs by BPMs (beats per minute) to add speed, and then create your own playlists. Although most people couldn't care less about BPMs, people in the fitness world are all about them because it's how we tailor our classes. BPMs are really only relevant to you when you're syncing music to the pace of your workout.

I know lots of people who love to listen to music when they're working. After a while it's just there, a wave to propel them along, a sonic backdrop that helps them do their tasks more efficiently. And, of course, music is the universal soother. It's why you sing lullabies to babies, or why you hear repetitive melodies when you're at a spa, about to have a massage. You'll start relaxing before you know it.

### Music Is Vibration

In 2000, I lived in India for two and a half months to study yoga. I went there at my friend Kelly's suggestion, as she was living there and loving how much yoga was bringing into her life. She could sense I was in need of a similar kind of change in *my* life, and I have her to thank for my amazing experiences with Pattabhi Jois in Mysore.

Even showing up was pretty crazy, though, because I had *never* taken even one yoga class, not anywhere. That didn't stop me from signing on at a center geared to yoga professionals, where everyone else had been doing yoga for, literally, decades. For each session, there would be anywhere from seventy-five to one hundred students at the *shala,* and at the end of each practice, there would be a chanting moment.

Well, I didn't know the chant, of course, because I'd never studied yoga before, and I was too inhibited to say that. So I listened to everyone else, and the only thing that got me through the chant, faking it till I was making it, was the fact that I had listened to Madonna's *Ray of Light* album so many times and I suddenly realized that the track "Ashanti" contained the actual chant my fellow yogis were saying at the end of class. It didn't take long before I found myself chanting the song instead of singing it. There I was, in that moment where art imitates life (thanks, Madonna!).

I soon realized that chanting—all kinds of singing, actually—is a form of vibration. What does that really mean? Well, your body is made up primarily of water, and it reacts to all the energy in the atmosphere and surroundings. According to quantum physics, everything in our universe is in constant motion—vibrating at specific frequencies. If, for example, I put a bottle of water on the podium during one of my classes, you'll see it vibrating from the bass in the songs I'm playing.

So your body will respond in its own way to different vibrations in music. I like to think of it as riding the music as if you were surfing; instead of tapping into the energy of the waves and the water underneath you, you're going to feel the swell of the rhythm, and it will literally propel you to keep moving.

Think of vibration this way: You know how you say some-times, "Whoa, that person has good vibes" . . . or the total op-posite, "Wow, that person has bad vibes"? That's because you are actually feeling the vibration of that person.

Even your own thoughts vibrate through your body, so you have to be super careful about what you're saying to yourself. You don't want to give your own body bad vibes! Speak nicely with that inner voice. It makes everything a whole lot better.

### *Moving Meditation Using Music to Energize You*

This needs to be done with your eyes closed, so make sure you're moving in a safe way, such as on a stationary bicycle, marching in place on a cushioned surface, or holding on tight with your hands on the treadmill.

---

SG TRUTH　I see people doing this on the treadmill all the time and think it's scary. Yikes! If you feel confident about it, just be super careful and go at a very slow pace.

---

1. Find yourself in the middle of one of your favorite songs, and surround yourself with rhythm. Time to become a better listener. Time to become a better, stronger, more confident *you*.
2. Close your eyes. Stay connected to your breath. I want you

to feel who you are on a cellular level with your eyes closed. This is *very* important. You can do it, but you have to trust.

3. Keep your eyes closed as you focus on the music and focus on *you*. There may come a time one day where you're going to be forced to keep your eyes closed and you're not going to be in the mood (cue MRI sound). When that happens, you'll be able to channel this moment, right here, right now, because you practiced closing your eyes when you were in control. Just breathe here. Focus on the timing of your feet and the presence of your mind inside your body. This moment is just about your movement and, simply, your breath.

4. Whatever you're going for in your life, whatever you're trying to achieve, *bring it*. Go for it today, right now. Visualize what you want. You'll get it—all you have to do is put the action behind the thought. Everything in this universe starts with your thoughts, and then the action comes to life after you put those thoughts into physical motion. Don't stop thinking about what you want. This is your moment right here. Walk yourself down the mental steps of what you need to do to put that thought into action. Maybe it's a phone call, a conversation, a text, an e-mail. Imagine yourself doing it, and then when you finish this meditation, go do it!

5. As the music winds down, stay in your Moving Meditation until you feel ready to stop. Do not forget to go. Put it into motion *now*. . . . *Go*!

⚜

# THE POWER OF NO IN THE NOW

So many of my students have told me about what happens when they finally say yes. Yes to the new job. Yes to the new beau. Yes to the dress.

Of course *yes* is a powerful word, but so is *no*. By saying no to things that aren't aligned with your intentions and goals, you are reinforcing and making space for what is important to you. Saying no to the things that take away from your goals creates space for them and tells the universe you are focused on them.

"Saying no can be very empowering."

Because women, in particular, are programmed early on to be more docile than men—for fear of being called pushy, overbearing, or selfish—even though, of course, they're not (and a man would never be called any of those words!)—they often have a hard time saying *no*. We are just conditioned to live in the House of Yes. But we still need to spend time in the House of No. It is important to know what you need to say yes to (the things you need to do to achieve your goals) and what you need to say no to (the things that are wasting your time or taking away from those goals).

When setting your intentions and defining your goals, and when used in the right context and for the right purpose, no can be very empowering. Especially if you *aren't* used to saying it. It is a firm statement and an acknowledged choice that gives you a jolt of adrenaline (which is a potent appetite suppressant, by the way).

It also means you're fully engaged in the *now*.

I've found that many of my students have a difficult time saying no. It's an avoidance technique that allows them to put off being honest about what they really want if they think it's going to upset someone. There's that fear that someone's going to react in a bad way and that you're going to have to deal with the repercussions of their anger; plus, you don't want to make people upset . . . so you say yes so they're not upset and you end up unraveling something in your day to compensate for having to take care of someone else's needs rather than your own.

That said, there's often a fine line to walk to ensure you're saying no for a valid reason. You might not want to say no, but logistically, it's just impossible to say yes. If so, try saying, "I might not be able to get to it today, but how about tomorrow?" Or "I can't do *this,* but how about I help you with *that?*"

The answer is still no in the now, but makes clear that you are available according to both of your schedules. You're offering alternatives, sort of the way you'd give a stubborn child the choice of three shirts to wear in the morning instead of saying, "No, you can't wear that."

Use *your* no to give someone else a choice—because what you want to avoid is falling into the trap of saying yes to please someone else, and then creating chaos in your own life as a result. This can quickly veer into martyr mode, where you're doing things out of a sense of obligation and using that to avoid dealing with *your* needs and *your* goals. My theory is to manage both the answer yes and the answer no, without feeling guilty about either!

## How Saying (or Not Saying) No Ties in to the Lies We All Tell

After years of addiction, I finally reached a tipping point. I knew that if I stayed in the place I was, physically and mentally, not only would have I become even more stuck in a self-destructive cycle, but something bad could have happened. Not only was my common sense screaming at me to get out of my toxic lifestyle, but my gut was throbbing so much it was like having my own internal drum kit.

I had to say no to my entire lifestyle. And I had to say no to all the lying.

I left my home, my family, my friends, my successful career to discover what it was like not to live in lies. When you're an addict, you lie every day. So your no is actually what's keeping you going. No was my denial about everything in my life.

I learned very quickly that it can be difficult to be an honest person. Not only was it easy for me to lie, but it was *comfortable* because I grew up lying, as you know. I lied to my classmates about my family situation and my parents being divorced because I was ashamed. And I lied about being gay. Back in the 1980s when I was growing up, there were no gay people my age. I was wearing my friend's boys' underwear underneath my clothes in fifth grade. Now it's trendy—but I shudder to think what my classmates would have said had they found out back then. No way could I have dealt with it, and, of course, no child should have to worry about such complicated matters, either.

The tightrope of truth is very hard to walk, but your life is so much better when you tell the truth. There may be more discomfort at first when you are honest, but secret-keeping is toxic and can literally make you sick.

And this gets back to setting your intentions and identifying your goals. If you can't be honest with yourself—even uncomfortably so—then what is the point? One of the hardest things we can ever do is confront our raw selves, with all our flaws and accomplishments, and see who we really are. Once you can do that, you are on your way toward attaining whatever it is you want.

## PUSHING PAST PROCRASTINATION

Are you still having trouble setting your intentions and defining your goals? Be honest—are you procrastinating? If so, I feel your pain!

For years, I was a world-class procrastinator. Dealing with adult responsibilities and paying my bills? Forget it. I had the worst credit of anyone I knew, and was basically drowning in off-the-books debt. I never paid any bills, and I owed friends and family money. I basically took forever to pay them back. I didn't have any credit cards; I asked to be paid in cash for all my gigs and spent the money as soon as it came in. I put off whatever I could. I was running in place. And I used my procrastination as an excuse not to make the changes I knew I needed to make.

Now it's the complete opposite. All my bills get paid the day they arrive, even if they aren't due for weeks. I've set up auto-pay for most of them, too, so I don't have to worry about being late. I can't stand owing anyone anything, and my credit is crazy good. But it took me *years* to catch up.

As I was transforming myself from a bill-avoiding slacker into a grown-up, I realized how much my procrastination had wasted years of my life. I was on the train, looking ahead to the tracks stretching out to the future, but I was stuck at the station. I had to get it together and *deal*.

Typically, the cycle of procrastination starts when whatever we have to do is daunting for some reason. It could be that you're lacking the energy to do it, or it could be fear-based or shame-based. Or you could just not feel like doing something. I mean, really, who wants to do the paperwork for their taxes, or wax the car, or clean out their overflowing e-mail inbox? But you have to look at those tasks as steps toward reaching your bigger goals.

One of the problems now for procrastinators is that social media and our digital lifestyle are thumbing their noses at you. They make it so easy to pretend you're doing things when you're scrolling through your Instagram feed. Before there were search engines, if you had to research something, you knew you had to block off the time to get to the library, riffle through the card catalog, find the book, read through the book, and write notes by hand. Now you can do that in a nano-flash online, freeing up a lot more time for screwing around, right?

Procrastinators also tend to be late. Are *you* chronically late? If so, you're the kind of person who doesn't respect time. But time is something you *must* respect, because it's the one thing you can't ever change. You can reset your watch if you travel to another time zone, but you cannot change the real time. And you can't change your chronological age. You can have a plastic surgeon make you look younger, but your body is still going to age. You're on the clock, you're born, you grow, and you die. Just be on time!

My mom, as an early riser, had late-person anxiety; she was always the first person to arrive anywhere. I followed in her footsteps and was the first kid at school and the last one to leave. I used to get upset by other people's lateness, but eventually I realized that it was their issue, not mine, and that people explain their lateness in different ways. Some are procrastinators who find every excuse not to get going.

Some like the power it gives them by making others wait for them. Some honestly don't like or feel comfortable with idle chatter, so they show up late for events so they don't have to worry about talking to others. Some are late because it honestly doesn't bother them—they're the last to board an airplane. That will *never* be me! If I'm late to a social event, it's only because I don't drink, so I typically skip cocktail hour.

I also realized that when it comes to procrastination, there are three types of people: people who wake up with no alarm, people who use the snooze button but don't really need it, and people who keep hitting snooze over and over and as a result are chronically late.

---

**SG TRUTH**    I set my alarm so that I have fifteen minutes to slowly wake up. In my head, I begin the conversation about what my day looks like, even though I'm still half asleep!

---

I figured this out because for the last few years, I have woken up at six fifteen A.M. without an alarm; I set it anyway just in case, as I teach a class at seven thirty and can't be late. Even if I didn't teach, I'd still wake up. I hear a certain truck rumbling down the street, and the cars on the nearby avenue, and I know it's time to get up.

So when my alarm goes off, I hit the snooze button, knowing that I have eight minutes to lie there, eyes closed, taking my time and going over my schedule in my head, until the alarm goes off again. I also know that I have forty-five minutes until I have to *really* leave—which means I could hit the snooze button five more times if I felt like it. But I don't. I like my routine. When the alarm goes off the second time, I am ready to get up and start my day.

If you're not in control of the snooze, it's going to control you. That's when I call it Chasing the Eight. (As in pool, not the snooze button!) When you play pool, the last ball you want to hit in the pocket is the eight ball—so during the entire game, you're chasing it so you can win. Sure, you're craving the extra sleep, but how much better is it to wake up, hit the ball in, and start your day? Chasing the eight ball with intention means you are ready to do the work *now,* do the workout *now,* finish the task *now.*

## How to Stop Procrastinating

Like any behavior you want to change, you start by setting your intentions. The mantra should be, "The motivated side is way better than this side. I have to do this. I know I can. It's way better on the motivated side. I am going to power up and get motivated."

My favorite tip for doing this is to use an old-fashioned egg timer.

Even though I was a terrible procrastinator about really important things when I lived in Los Angeles, I never put off the house cleaning. Because I have a mild form of what I think is OCD, I just loved getting obsessive with dusting and tidying—it was super satisfying because I could see immediate results. This made my roommate at the time, Chuck, crazy because I was always cleaning. So he'd set the egg timer for an hour, and the rule was I had to stop as soon as it went off. That got me into the very useful habit of blocking off my time to get things done, even the unpleasant ones. Simply set the timer, and force yourself to stop procrastinating when it goes off.

I find that it helps to block out a specific amount of time where your task will fit. When you set your alarm for that task, whatever it is, remind yourself in the block *before* it that this task is coming up. That way, you can start preparing yourself to start wrapping up what's in the first block so that by the time you get to the second block, you're golden.

For example, all my classes are fifty minutes long, yet there are always students who leave early. Not only is it disruptive for my concentration and rude to the other riders, but it takes all the joy out of the late shift's rides because they're going to be more worried about the clock than about focusing on the workout. *Why*, I ask them, are you backing up appointments so close to this class that you have to leave early? Why aren't you better at managing your time blocks?

If you're leaving to get to work on time, it means you're inviting your boss into my class, and he's not allowed in there. And quite frankly, I don't know one boss in New York City who wouldn't be lenient if you told him that you have a class where you train really hard in the mornings, and that you're willing to cut down on your lunch hour or stay an extra fifteen minutes later at the end of the day so you could finish your class without rushing and worrying about being late. Because after a hard training session, your brain is going to be on fire, and you'll be bringing so much more to the office. You're working out not just for you, but because you want to be the best team player possible.

A lot of times, getting over procrastination just means you need a jolt of energy to get you over that first hurdle. If so, set the egg timer for a minute or two and do twenty jumping jacks, or as many as you can until the timer goes off. This will get the blood flowing and your brain stimulated. Just *jump*. Then take a deep breath, jump in the shower, get ready for your task, and do it. You know how good you're going to feel when the task is done, and then of course you'll wonder why you kept putting it off.

It's like that feeling you get when you finally clean out your out-of-control closet. I know how the feeling of where to start can feel paralyzingly overwhelming . . . and then when you're in the middle of making the piles of clothing you wonder when you'll ever finish . . . and then at the end, when you have bags of items to donate and you can see the closet floor for the first time in ages, suddenly, you've never felt better. Even your *thoughts* are clearer!

Key to all of this is to focus on the end result *before* you start. That will keep you going, and going, and going.

# FIVE
## CREATING
## SPACE FOR
## CHANGE

Once you've set your intentions and goals for a healthier life-style, there is one more thing you need to do before you start. In the next part of the book, I'm going to take you through my LET program, but first you need to get in the mood to crush it. And the way to do that, believe it or not, is to clean up your house. And your car, and your garage. You're going to get moving to do this. Think of all the calories you'll be burning while you get rid of stuff that is weighing you down. It's a win-win, believe me!

"If you have clutter everywhere, you're telling the universe your thoughts are a jumbled-up mess."

## CLEAR YOUR CLUTTER

Clutter clearing is not the same thing as creative visualization, but as a tool it's just as important. (Trust me on this: I've never heard of anyone stepping over clutter in a visualization—your mind knows how unnecessary it is!) The mental task of deciding what to keep or not, and the physical task of picking it up and figuring out whether to give it away, throw it away, or recycle it lightens your load.

What you surround yourself with is extremely important to your ability to lose weight and keep it off and to improve your overall well-being. How you feel about yourself and your body is reflected in your home, car, and office. If you have clutter everywhere, you're telling the universe your thoughts are a jumbled-up mess. If your house is dirty, you are telling the universe you don't respect your living space. If you buy clothes you know you'll never wear and your closets are filled to bursting, you're telling the universe you're filling a void that is replacing your common sense.

---

**SG TRUTH**   I have way too many things. I need to do this myself, believe me, and I do it often but not enough. I have clothes *everywhere,* in every closet, on every rolling rack in my office, everywhere. But it is 90 percent organized, and there is always room to improve. . . . My girlfriend is asking me in this very moment to get a pair of my sneakers out of her office. Believe me, the cleanup never ends!

---

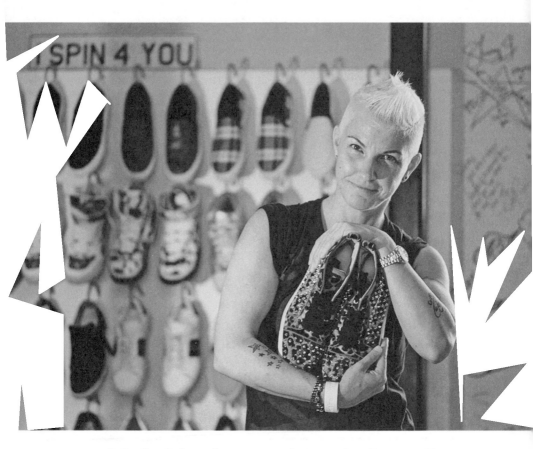

I absolutely love clearing my clutter—when I eventually get to it. I know that part isn't easy. You have to schedule the time like a doctor's appointment—and not cancel on yourself! I finally got around to the long-overdue clear-out thanks to my mentor, Tony Robbins. And yes, I'm the first to admit that my closets have been known to get a bit too full and my shoe collection takes up several walls in my office.

This task should not fill you with anxiety. Please don't think of it as me telling you to get rid of everything. I'm not asking you to be in denial about or erase your past, or to be defensive about the reasons that led you to buy or obtain certain items. I've held on to plenty of things that I'll never wear or use, but since they were given to me by someone important, I cherish them for their sentimental value. Maybe I'll keep all of them, or maybe I'll keep just a few.

I was reminded of this when, one day, a friend's seven-year-old looked at the pile of all the drawings she'd done in her life—the huge pile her mother had kept because she loved all of them—and asked her mom, "Why do you have *all* of them? Some of them are really bad! Throw them away!" This child was a better editor of her own work than her mother would ever be. She didn't feel the need to keep something just because she'd done it. What a smart little girl!

When you're getting ready to start a decluttering session, find a slot where you won't be interrupted. You don't want to have to rush, as that's when you'll accidentally throw something out you meant to keep or just get fed up or frustrated and quit in the middle. I suggest that you start small and take it slow.

Focus on one area at a time. Don't expect to clear the clutter all at once. Get out your trusty egg timer and set it for ten minutes at first. Stop when it dings.

Keep going, in ten-minute increments, if you have the momentum and are able to be honest and ruthless. If not, fix a date for the next session and set the timer for fifteen minutes for that session. It's much easier to handle this kind of task when you know it will be over soon or that you can do it in small sessions.

Be prepared for how you're going to feel. Clutter clearing is extremely empowering, but it can also trigger a lot of memories and the painful kind of thinking this book will help you leave behind, things like "Why did I waste so much money on this dress?" or "Was I ever this skinny?" The goal should be to look at your clutter and say, "I know somebody else really needs it and will love wearing this coat I never wore," or "I am going to buy nice new clothes that fit me perfectly and enhance my figure *now*." Whatever the internal dialogue you choose, make sure you stay positive with the affirmations, and never forget that *you* are your biggest cheerleader!

Ultimately, what I want you to do is fall out of love with your unnecessary possessions, and fall in love with what really matters.

For today, let's start with the kitchen, because that's where the food is.

## How to Do a Kitchen Cleanse

The only way to have the healthy, strong body you want is by eating the right foods. If the foods you can't resist are sitting on your pantry shelves, you're going to eat them when the cravings hit. So let's get cleansing.

First, get some large trash bags, some large recycling bags, and some large cardboard boxes.

SG TRUTH   In our fridge at home we have things "on tap" like blueberries, raspberries, strawberries, bananas, oranges, pineapple, sliced watermelon, and lots of water. They're right there on every shelf when you open the door so all your eyes see are healthy choices. In the cupboard drawers we have carbs like dark pretzels and granola bars, so there's always something grab-able and good for us.

*Ditch these into the trash:*
- All food that's expired.
- All stale dried herbs and spices (anything you've had for longer than a year that's lost its potency—sniff or taste the herb or spice if you're not sure).
- All frozen food that's been in the freezer longer than six months or has passed its best-by date. At the very least, it'll have freezer burn and will not taste good.

*Place these in the boxes for donation to your local food pantry, because you know there's nothing worse than wasting food, even if it isn't very healthy:*
- All unexpired dry/canned goods that you forgot about or know you won't eat.
- All packaged junk food.

*Recycle:*
- Any empty bottles or containers that you bought or kept for storage but never actually used.

*Replace with:*
- Nutritious food.

Clean out the refrigerator and defrost the freezer while you're at it. Rearrange your pantry or cabinet shelves by category (grains on one shelf, legumes on another, etc.). Place the less-used or unhealthy items like flour and sugar on high shelves so you won't see them when you open the cabinets.

## How to Do a Closet Cleanse

Next, move on to your clothes and shoes, closets and drawers. It's tough to be ruthless because there is often a sentimental attachment to articles of clothing. That's okay. You can keep items that are important to you. Just not *all* of them!

As with food, get large trash bags and boxes.

*Ditch these into the trash, cut them up for use as rags, or set them aside as playthings for your kids:*
- Anything that's torn, stained, falling apart, and/or beyond repair.
- Underwear, bras, and swimsuits that have lost their elasticity or support, and orphan socks.

*Remove these and place in bags or boxes for donation\* (be sure to ask for receipts, as donations are tax deductible):*

- Anything that never fit and never will.
- Anything that reminds you of a bad time in your life.
- Anything that isn't your style but was so expensive/bought on a whim/was super-marked down and the best bargain of your life so you fell for it anyway. If you've never worn it, it wasn't a bargain even if it was 90 percent off!
- Anything you've worn only once, even if you still like it.
- Anything you haven't worn in the last year, unless it has sentimental value and/or is a special-occasion item you know you're going to need for your nephew's wedding in a few months.

\*For high-ticket items, consignment shops will pay you when the items sell. There are even online consignment sites likes Vestiaire that make the selling extremely easy, no matter where you live. Charities like Goodwill or shelters are always in need. No matter what you paid for it, clothing you donate will always be worth more to someone who can actually use it. This is also one of those good-karma moments in your life. Give it away!

*Keep these:*

- Clothing and shoes you wear all the time.
- Clothing and shoes you wear for special events so you don't have to buy anything new. (Panic buying usually leads to never-gonna-wear-it-after-all mistakes!)

- Your grandmother's favorite cashmere sweater, even though it doesn't fit and it's so out of style you'd never wear it in public.
- Special-occasion clothes you rarely wear but need to have (formal wear, a business suit if you work in a nonbusiness job, etc.).
- One item in your goal size, if and only if that helps you. For some people, having a wonderful article of clothing in the closet as Goal Pants or a Goal Little Black Dress is a great motivator—because losing the weight and finally wearing it is proof of your hard work and dedication. If that's not you, get rid of it!

*Replace with:*

- Clothing and shoes that fit you now, are comfortable, stylish, and make you feel good. When you lose weight, you can have too-large items fixed. Here's a fashion tip—practically any article of clothing can be altered by a good tailor. Smart women save a bundle by buying nondesigner clothes and having them tailored. It's amazing how much better clothing looks when it fits you perfectly. Don't forget that the donation sites for couture clothing also sell things! So if you're looking for something high end, start there first before you head to the department store. You may find an expensive item at 70 percent off.

---

SG TRUTH   I finally caved and hired a closet organizer. She saved me about two full days of cleaning and tossing anything I didn't feel I could "release." If you can afford a professional organizer to help you, do it. He or she will have zero attachment to any of your things and will help you make smart choices you're unable to face on your own. It will be money well spent!

---

## How to Do a Bathroom Cleanse

Now that you have nice, organized closets and drawers, it's time to move on to the room many people ignore. Instead of looking at your bathroom as a space you *need* to use, consider it as a space you *want* to use—your sanctuary. It's kind of hard to have your own Spiritual Bath space if the shelves are lined with yucky old nearly empty bottles of shampoo!

*Ditch these:*

- The scale. I never weigh myself. I don't need to and you don't, either. Weight fluctuates so much that constant (especially daily) weighing can truly impede your weight-loss progress, and I have always monitored my weight by how well my clothes fit. (For the record, I weigh 143 pounds and am usually a size 6.) You should do the same.

  Muscle weighs more than fat, so if you're working out a lot more than in the past, you might weigh the same but actually have dropped several sizes and lowered your BMI, or Body

Mass Index. *That's* what counts. The way your clothes fit your body is all that matters. This is the best way to keep on top of yourself. You don't want to get bigger than your clothes— and if you do, please go to your physician for a physical. (You might have a thyroid condition or something else going on that could be affecting your metabolism. This is especially important if you have any sudden weight gain or loss.) And, if you still feel the need to see that number, hide the scale in the back of your closet, inside a suitcase, and weigh yourself no more than once a month.

- Beauty products you don't use or never liked. As with clothing, you can have a cabinet full of items that might have looked good when the salesperson talked you into forking over the cash, but they don't suit you. If they're unopened, donate them to your local shelter. If not, toss it out, or donate it with your clothing (this is safe to do as long as you ditch any applicators and wipe any lipsticks with an alcohol-saturated tissue. The only exceptions are mascara and eye liner—these should be thrown out).

- Beauty items that have expired. Powders last longer than creamy products. Sunscreen expires after about a year, even though the packaging might say up to three years. Check the box or bottle carefully.

*Replace with:*

- Items that entice all your senses. I love my SB by SG bath products and use them every day. I also have my scented candles near the bath, and thick towels. My bath time is my time to unwind. Your bathroom should be a haven, not just a place to brush your teeth and poop.

## How to Clear Your Living Room/Family Room

Many people have rooms with way too much stuff in them. Move things around so there is a clear flow of energy. I often suggest that you use this room for exercising, because there should be a TV or a table where you can set up a computer so you can do your workouts to music and/or along with a professional teacher/coach/trainer on the screen, and you'll have space to move around. You need to choose a room where you're most likely to do the workouts easily, without distractions. You also need a portable box filled with exercise bands, small hand weights, and a nonskid yoga mat for padding.

*Ditch these:*

- Furniture that's broken, stained, or not comfortable anymore.
- Small items like vases and souvenirs that are just gathering dust.

*Keep these:*

- What you love, what you use, and what's comfortable. Donate the rest, as long as it's in good condition.

## How to Do a Garage/Basement/Attic Cleanse

Many of my fellow New Yorkers don't have to worry about excess clutter in attics or garages, as they live in apartments far smaller than many homes outside of the city. Most buildings charge for storage, too, which limits how much stuff you can accumulate. It's amazing to realize how much you don't need when you know you have to pay a large monthly fee to store it!

If you do have an attic, basement, and/or garage, they can be ideal spots for the clutter you know you should get rid of—but don't *have* to because you have the space to hide it away. Don't let this be an excuse, because having nice clean and empty spaces atop and below where you live is wonderfully freeing. Clutter is heavy energy. You need clear channels all around you!

*Ditch these:*

- Anything you don't need.
- Anything in a box that's been there for so long you couldn't even remember what it was and why you saved it.
- Broken tools and half-empty containers of decades-old antifreeze or paint.

---

**SG TRUTH** Now that there is a wallet on my cell phone with a thumbprint code, an Uber app where you don't need cash to pay for a ride, and Apple Pay at most stores, leaving your wallet at home doesn't have the worst repercussions—but leaving your phone does! Ha!

---

I'm the kind of person who just plunges into a swimming pool, so I used to playfully chide the double-checkers—you know, those who have to test the water temperature first and then take twenty minutes to finally get in. But then I got over myself when I realized they had a system, and that I was the one who needed a system for all the things I was forgetting to double-check. Like what was in my wallet and pockets and bag when I left the house and then realized I'd forgotten something essential. Like, um, my *keys*.

What I finally figured out was that you need to clear the clutter to alleviate chaos before you leave. It's the only way you can follow through with your intentions and have peace. Believe me, if you're hours away from home and realize you don't have your house keys, you are not going to have a peaceful moment until you figure out what to do!

So what I've seared into my brain is my leaving-the-house High Five. (A friend of mine calls this the Idiot Check—as in, if you forget anything, you're the idiot!) Keys, wallet, cell phone, charger, smile. Five items so I can High Five myself.

You might have a High Three or a High Eight—but whatever else is on your checklist, the smile is the most important. Even more so than your keys. Because your smile is your intention. You have everything you need for the day. Acknowledge your intention, and smile in gratitude for the brain that has drawn up your MAP to get you motivated and your body that is in motion.

## How to Do a Car Cleanse

Is your car a mess? Why? Would you be mortified if your boss asked for a ride home and saw the clutter and empty fast-food boxes and empty soda or water bottles tossed in the backseat? Or what if you went on a job interview and the person in charge of hiring you got a good look at the mess—do you think you would get the job? I don't think so.

I think about this a lot, as my mom was in sales her whole life. She was really good at it. She knew that her car needed to be immaculate because she might potentially have just made the biggest sale of her life with Mr. X, and what would she do if Mr. X suddenly asked her for a ride home? She knew that the second Mr. X got in her car, she would be judged. Messy car = messy person = no sale. Who wants to do business with someone who doesn't care about their environment? My mom's car was always in impeccable shape.

Be like my mom—keep your car washed and polished and the inside detailed. You want your car to be as sparkling as you'd want it to be if Ryan Gosling asked you for a ride home.

*Ditch these:*
- Any food items.
- Any dirty containers.
- Empty or half-full water or soda bottles.
- Anything that doesn't belong in a car, such as a bag of old gym clothes or sports equipment, empty roadie cups, chipped coffee mugs, maps that are falling apart, broken

umbrellas, extra forks and knives from last year's picnic—all of which have been in my car at some point!

*Replace with:*

- A small bottle of sunscreen, as you can get a nasty sunburn without realizing it while driving.
- Hand sanitizer for those messy moments.
- A chamois and dust-brush for spot-cleaning.

*Cleaning out your car is a great workout. Vacuum the inside and wash the mats. Wash the outside and then polish it. Your arms and abs will thank you.

# PLAYLIST
## FOR CLEARING OUT THE CLUTTER

Use these songs as a soundtrack to your clutter clearing. Nothing like a little dance party to keep you upbeat as you sort through the piles! These are all sing-alongs, which is the point. You want to whistle while you work!

| | |
|---|---|
| Beyoncé | "Formation" |
| Tracy Chapman | "Fast Car" |
| Chuva Speaks Arab | "Reckless Girl" |
| Eminem | "Cleaning Out My Closet" |
| David Guetta ft. Usher | "With or Without You" |
| Quinton Harris-Koffee | "Paradise" |
| HiPOST | "Livin' It Up by Jagged Edge" |
| Bruno Mars | "Uptown Funk" |
| Ben Pearce | "What I Must Do" |
| TLC | "No Scrubs" |

## PRIME YOUR BODY FOR CHANGE: FIRST, CLEAR THE CLUTTER OUT OF YOUR BODY

One day, not that many years ago, I was talking with Meredith Geller, my holistic nutrition consultant, about cravings. Namely, my insatiable cravings for chewy candy like Red Vines and licorice. Those cravings had started when I was doing a lot of drugs and needed a sugar rush when I was coming down off a bender so I could get up and go teach a class with my usual pep with none of my students the wiser. After I got clean, my cravings for chewy candy didn't diminish. If anything, they got worse.

"Hmm," she said as I told her all this. "Do you know what you're really eating when you eat candy like that?"

"Nope," I said, chewing on another Red Vine.

"*Plastic*," she replied.

I stopped chewing. "What? What do you mean, plastic?"

"They're not just made of a lot of sugar. They also have a lot of the same chemicals found in different plastics. Just so you know."

I looked at the shiny bag of candy. "You're kidding me, right?" I said, hoping she was just saying that to stop me from scarfing it down.

"I wish I were," Meredith replied. "Just think about that next time you find your hand in a bag of candy. Say to yourself: 'It's *plastic*.'" She waited for a beat, then added, "And you know what plastic is, too, don't you? It's *poison*. Nonbiodegradable, indigestible *poison*. Got it?"

Well, that was an OMG moment. I thanked her, threw the bag in the garbage, and have tried really, really hard not to eat them anymore.

---

**SG TRUTH**   Do I still have them occasionally? Yes, but I don't buy them every day anymore. Believe me, I used to eat candy *every* day!

---

My association with the sweet treats I once loved so much has been so tainted that I can't think of any candy without seeing my intestines all twisted up and clogged with little beads of plastic. Talk about a deterrent!

The pathway to radiance and good health starts with a solid foundation and an unraveling of built-up toxicity. This foundation is laid when you cleanse your body. Think of it as clearing the clutter from your system.

To create harmony, longevity, beauty, radiance, vibrancy, and true wellness from the inside out, we need to follow basic principles of the laws of nature. This will allow your body to be the brightest expression of itself on every level.

I love cleansing. (Meredith told me that using the word *cleanse* as a noun is actually incorrect—you want to think of this process as a verb.) I knew that my liver and pancreas are the organs in my body responsible for detoxification, but thanks to the kind of food most of us eat and our polluted environment and all the stresses of modern life, they needed extra help. That means cleansing is an ongoing process. Cleansing comes in many different forms—it can be from fasting, mono-diets (eating one food only for a few days), juicing, drinking bone broth, or others. Obviously, not everyone likes or can tolerate certain types of cleansing, and of course you should never start a period of cleansing without consulting your physician and/or certified nutritionist or advisor, who can tailor it to your needs. I also recommend that you do it in stages, start-

## HOW TO DO A BODY CHECK

Be sure to get a comprehensive checkup with your physician as well as a full blood work-up before you start any weight-loss or workout regimen. This is common sense, but I'm always shocked when my students tell me they haven't seen a doctor for years. You can be surprisingly deficient in certain vitamins or minerals, especially vitamin D; you might also have hormonal imbalances, especially with your thyroid; you might also have blood sugar issues. These can affect your progress and make it very difficult to lose weight or have normal energy levels. I learned this the hard way. I've always been a chronic ice chewer—I could tell you the name of every restaurant in my neighborhood that has great ice! One savvy doctor asked me if I had this habit and told me it was a symptom of anemia (go figure!) and ordered immediate blood tests. Turns out I was severely anemic (levels are measured at 1–500 and mine was 13) and could have gotten very, very sick. I suffered from a lot of totally avoidable problems for years because I avoided getting a checkup. Don't let that be you!

ing with gentle, short cleansing periods and then working up to more intense, longer plans.

The "cleaner" we eat and the better care we take in feeding our bodies, the more potent all the nutrients we ingest will be. Everything in the body functions better when it is lighter and clearer.

## TRAIN YOUR MOUTH

Eating isn't like exercise in just one respect: You can get through life without ever doing a proper workout (not that anyone should!), but you can't get through more than a few days without food and water. Just as you know that the key to success with fitness and everything else is to keep moving, every day of your life, the key to success with food is training your mouth. You can do this just as you train your muscles every time you exercise.

The following steps will show you what to do.

### Recognize That Change Doesn't Happen Overnight

If you move two steps backward and one step forward, no biggie. Just make sure that the one forward step is bigger than the two backward ones. It took me many tries to stop drinking over many years—but I finally did. And *many* years to stop drugging, but it eventually stuck forever!

You didn't put weight on overnight, either. I always tell the moms who come to my classes that it took nine months for them to nurture their babies inside their bodies, and they should set a nine-month goal to lose the weight. Chances are you will lose it in far less time than nine months, but the target date should be nine months from the day your baby was born. If you get there early, congratulate yourself. You made a human! Or if it takes a little longer, that's okay, too, because at least you have a reference point to know you should be on your way back to "you."

## Clear the Clutter in Your Head About Food

Now that you've cleared the clutter from your house, it's time to clear the clutter from your head.

Set your intentions about eating. This visualization is one of my favorites and will not let you down!

### Visualization for Dealing with Food Issues and/or Weight Loss: Think Orange

Use this visualization as a template whenever you need help focusing on issues about your weight and/or weight loss. This one is particularly useful whenever you feel the need for encouragement. Do it before you have to go to dinner at your in-laws', where too much food is always piled on your plate by your sabotaging relatives. Do it before a company picnic where there will be loads of your favorite foods. Do it before you to go the movies, when all you want is a big bag of buttered popcorn and a bag of candy, washed down with a supersized soda. (I always get a small popcorn without butter and a bottle of water.)

Do it before you go to the grocery store, where you're tempted to buy the wrong things.

1. Go to a quiet place where you won't be disturbed and where you can sit or lie down comfortably. Close your eyes, breath deeply and steadily throughout.

2. Focus on the color orange. Everything you are going to see will be orange. You have splashed an entire canvas with orange paint. This color fills your eyes and your senses. It is bright, glowing. It is the color of power and resolve.

3. Keep thinking orange. The success of all your issues with your weight is about getting focused on them, acknowledging them, and ridding them from your life.

4. Try *listening* to the color orange. That's right. (No, it's not crazy!) Breathe in, breathe out. Through your ears is the focus here. That's what listening is. You're listening now to a color that you're seeing with your eyes. (This is teaching you intense concentration and patience.)

5. Open your eyes and go about your day. Remember that when you put yourself into that situation where there's food you know isn't good for you, you don't have to say yes when people offer it to you. Keep your water in one hand and your cell phone in the other if you have a hard time.

Stop using negative words toward yourself. No more "I wish I had," "I shouldn't have," "I can't believe I did that," "Why didn't I do this?," "I'm so stupid," "What was I thinking?"

Replace them with a new playlist. Instead, write down and say positive mantras all day, every day. (You can get some from my app 2 Turns from Zero.) Put Post-it notes on the doors and mirrors and refrigerator. I do this all the time. My all-time favorite is *Crush It!*

If you like, you can reinforce your eating goals with photographs—role-model photographs of a fit and healthy adult with strong muscles. Someone like Serena Williams, Gabby Reece, Michelle Obama, or another athlete or accomplished woman you respect.

No more self-punishment, okay? No one ever makes perfect choices all the time and eats a perfect diet every day—if they did, they'd be missing out on some of the most delicious pleasures in life. Nobody is a perfect eater, and it's impossible to be one. It's not normal, and no one expects you to do that. Just eat smart. I know you can. I mean, I try to eat the healthiest diet possible, but I don't always. What a bore it would be if I never had another french fry at Fred's on Sunday, or a slice of birthday cake, or, yes, even my number one craving, Red Vines.

Stop beating yourself up if you eat a cupcake. You are not a failure because you got a sugar craving. Do not assume that because you ate a bag of potato chips, you've permanently derailed your eating plan and you'll never lose weight. Balance that mistake with a double workout that day or the next day—think of it as calories on, calories off.

You're aiming for the center, remember? As my ninety-seven-year-old grandma calls it: "The Middle!" There are foodie fascists on one end, rolling their eyes at the thought of eating anything other than an artisan slice of hearth-baked spelt bread topped with Russian kale they grew themselves from seeds, and the junk-food junkies on the other, their fingers stained orange from the Cheez-Its they snatched out of their third-grader's lunch box. You, I am certain, fall somewhere in the middle!

Ban the word *cheating* from your vocabulary. When you tell yourself you cheated, it means that your mind is in the wrong place. You are setting yourself up to view food as good (perfect, unattainable diet) and bad (fast food, sugar, trigger foods you secretly binge on). Food isn't good or bad. It is nourishment.

Shake it off. When punishing words or self-flagellation rear up despite your best efforts, you need to kick them to the curb. Give yourself a shake-it-off moment. Find a buzzword that means something to you. It can be "Hey!" or "Yo!" or even just the word *pivot*. It should be positive, with energy and love attached to it. Then go into a room where you'll have privacy, and jump up and down (or march in place) while saying that buzzword. Trust me, this works. Before you know it, the punishment words and the cravings disappear.

Snack well. Grab a walnut and crack it and eat it, or a celery stick stack, or drink some cold, cold water. All these options help.

⚜

## Ask Yourself If You're Really and Truly Hungry

People often eat mindlessly because they're bored. Or unhappy. Or procrastinating. Eating gives you something to do in the moment. It tastes yummy. It's a distraction. It can temporarily make you feel good. But it can never be a replacement for admitting to what you're feeling when you decide to eat instead.

Be honest. If you're really hungry, eat! If you're not, give yourself a *pivot,* as above, or do a Moving Meditation or Visualization.

## Urge Surf Your Cravings Away

I don't like the word *trigger* as it's used to refer to food cravings, because it's the kind of word that's jarring and puts fear in your mind. Much better to deal with cravings by Urge Surfing.

An Urge Surf is a visualization technique I learned from my addiction counselor. When you think about something that you know is not a good choice, that is not part of your ultimate plan, instead of succumbing to the bad choice, turn it into a wave. Allow it to be nothing more than a passing wave, and then surf through the urge and let it pass.

When you Urge Surf, I suggest you close your eyes, because that takes you outside your immediate surroundings. You don't see what's worrying you and making you want to eat a carton of ice cream. You just see the waves and surf through them. You could actually use this technique as a meditation if you want to, simply by placing your current thought inside the wave and letting it pass through you and onto the shore, releasing it from your body. Not a bad idea—try one now!

## Reward Yourself with Good Food and Atmosphere

Most people associate what they're eating with good and bad. This starts the first time a toddler is given a sweet dessert for eating all her mac and cheese and green beans.

But if you think of food = rewards = sweets or your favorite (nonhealthy) foods, then where does the punishment fit in? By allowing you to eat the wrong foods. After all, who rewards themselves by eating broccoli? Well, you do! Or, you *will,* once you've trained your mouth. When you do eat, enjoy it. Savor it. Be glad you are eating well. Take your time. Chew your food

Back when I was still addicted to plastic candy, I used to make cinnamon toothpicks. There's something about cinnamon that instantly zaps your appetite.

This is what you do: Take cinnamon oil, pour it in a zip-top bag, add the toothpicks, roll them around gently with your fingers to get them covered, dump them out on a paper towels, separate them, and let them dry. I'd keep them in a little jar, and when the cravings hit, I'd pop one in my mouth and suck on it. It worked every time!

MY FAVORITE APPETITE KILLER

instead of gobbling it down. Pleasure is so often overlooked when you're eating—but it is a vital part of learning to eat well.

This also means you should never save the "good china" for company only, as my mother used to do. You are just as worthy as the best company you'll ever entertain. Set a place at the table, even if (and *especially* if) you're on your own that night. Use a cloth napkin. Light candles if you like. Arrange the food artfully on the plate. Be aware of your surroundings and all the senses that are engaged when you smell something delicious and then taste it. The more delicious your food, the more satiating and satisfying it is, so you will automatically eat *less* of it.

## Train Your Eye, Too

Since super-sizing entered the fast-food realm, portion sizes across the board have increased to a ridiculous degree. A bottle of Coke used to have only six ounces inside—now you can get it in two *liters*! If you're used to a certain volume of food being a "normal" size, it's easy to underestimate how much you're actually eating. It's also very easy to overlook how many serving sizes are listed on food labels. A serving of chicken should be only as big as the palm of your hand, not cover the entire plate. A serving of pasta is only two ounces—not half the box.

Use these tricks to small-size your super-sizes:

- Eat with chopsticks. It is impossible to take big bites or eat fast with this handy utensil.

- Use smaller plates.
- Use smaller utensils.
- Eat half of what's on your plate. Really. Push it away or ask for it to be wrapped up if you're eating out. Give your stomach time to adjust to the volume of food you just ate. Chances are, you aren't still hungry—you just *think* you are.

## The Power of No in the Now—for Food

As you learned, the Power of No in the Now means you're not saying yes simply because someone else wants you to. With food, it means you are addressing the craving and that your willpower is stronger than that craving.

I have students who find themselves in the kitchen, opening the cabinets in search of an unhealthy snack, who then stand in the middle of room, give themselves a jolt, jump up and down a few times, shout out "NO!," and then leave the kitchen.

Doing regular exercises gives you muscle memory. Saying No in the Now gives you *mental* muscle memory. Once you know your no works, it gets easier and easier to say it and to stick to it.

If, for example, you're eating out with friends and someone offers you a taste of something, or orders a bunch of desserts for the entire table, don't get pissed off at them (especially if you think they're jealous of your determination to eat well and trying to undermine your evening out). Simply use this as an opportunity to practice No in the Now with what I call the One-Bite Technique. If you're longing to try something scrumptious and calorie dense, go right ahead. Have one bite. Appreciate it. Then say, "No, thank you, I've had enough." Because you know you have!

Saying No in the Now also means you're acknowledging what is going on in your head at precisely that moment in time. *Now* is such a powerful word. (Just ask Eckhart Tolle—he is the master of *now*.) You aren't thinking about what you ate yesterday and you aren't thinking about what you're going to eat tomorrow. This is a great focusing technique. It shuts off the "Why did I" and the "I'm going to" thoughts, and makes you deal with the situation at hand. Getting better at being fully present in the moment will help you in so many other aspects of your life, too.

Ready to move on? Great! I've given you the tools you need to set your intentions, and it's time to apply them to the most important situations we all deal with in life. In the rest of the book, I'll show you how to Love, Eat, Train, and Repeat. You're going to learn how to mean it when you do it, full of determination to change your life. You're going to go for it, right now, because today is a new day. You're going to finally believe that this is your universe, and you were born into it for a reason. You're here, you made it—now do something! Let's rock this universe together!

# PART III
# ACTION

"Easy doesn't change you."

# SIX
## LOVE

You might wonder what love has to do with living a healthier lifestyle, losing weight, and getting in shape. The fact is, the only way to truly come into your own and find your Ultimate Center is by loving yourself first. That means accepting your own power, forgiving yourself for your faults and mistakes, and acknowledging that you deserve to live a healthy life full of joy. That's what I did when I found my own healing through the power of exercise. Let me show you how to move toward more self-love and acceptance so you can radiate confidence, courage, and charisma, and fill your heart with joy.

I know it's not easy. In fact, it can be excruciatingly tough. The emotional component of life is something that most of us *don't* like to talk about. We'd rather just avoid talking about feelings in general when they involve vulnerability, intensity, sensitivity, pain, or anything uncomfortable. But because everything good you want to be and to have in life has to do with love, you have to figure out a way to talk about it. If you know you need a certain kind of love (romantic, professional, purpose, children, friendship) but you're not getting it, it's easy to fall into the trap of thinking you're undeserving or that something is wrong with you.

Typically, when one of my students is going through a rough time and not loving themselves, I can tell. I see it in their posture, I see it in the expression on their faces when a specific song comes on; I see it in the way they handle themselves in the stretch, when everyone else is energized and they are drooping with tension or sadness. Often I am secretly excited to watch a person change their entire being in a matter of minutes. I know I'm about to open a door for them that they can run through. I always believe I can do it for them—the question is, do *they*?

In general, the way you are feeling inside shows up on the way you look on the outside. If you have let your appearance slide— you're really not into the clothes you wear, you don't bother to look good, and you aren't making any plans for yourself socially—chances are you're in an emotional rut with yourself, as if you've given up on love . . . and it's time to get out.

But how? How do you mentally pull it together enough to make the changes you need in a way that makes you happy to

# SEXY
# STRONG
# CONFIDENT

be living your life, regardless of your circumstances (especially if they're stressful circumstances like job loss, a painful breakup or divorce, or the loss of a loved one), and to be able to look for the love you need or keep the love you have alive? How do you not let tough circumstances zap you of all your will and your desire to love?

I believe you can handle any life stress with an inspiring coach who believes in you (here I am!), the knowledge that you need to keep on moving, and a healthy way of eating. You already learned that in order to find your confidence level and your happiness, you have to have purpose. You have to have a reason to live. A reason to get up. A reason to believe in love.

Because love is there for you, whether you believe it or not.

## FIRST, LOVE YOURSELF

What is love? It's so many things to so many people. According to my trusty and well-thumbed dictionary, it's an "intense feeling of deep affection, warmth, intimacy, attachment, endearment." Love isn't just about romantic love—it encompasses all members of your family, especially your children if you have them; your friends; your passions; your pets; your causes; your hobbies; your home; and all the things that engage your senses, like music, art, books, the handwoven little rug you haggled over in a Turkish bazaar, your childhood teddy bear, the blooming peonies in your garden, the way fresh bread smells when it comes out of the oven.

Finding love can make you feel more alive, more exhilarated, more enchanted than practically anything else on earth. It makes you feel as if you've discovered your true authentic self. Losing it, on the other hand, is like losing everything you've ever known and cared about.

In order to attract and keep the love you want in your life, you need to start with one basic thing: *You must love yourself.*

The cliché of this is the one you already know . . . and that is you have to believe you are lovable in order for love to find you. I'm not saying be narcissistic; I'm saying you need to feel your inner mojo if you expect that someone else should, too!

Your family, your work, your friends, your partner—you only attract love in your life if you love yourself. Your vibe is what attracts your tribe to you. The vibration of *not* loving yourself is so negative, people won't want to be next to you—it's *that* powerfully subliminal—without you even having to say a word. You won't be putting out the kinetic energy that is like a leaf blower, sending it out into the universe. In fact, when you don't love yourself, your aura shifts. You lack vibration as opposed to having a strong one that people can feel when you walk into a room. Instead of exuding happy and enticing pheromones (which are chemicals all animals exude to try to change the behavior of others in their species), you're wafting out what I call fear-o-mones.

Believe me, I know how hard it is to give off the love-myself/ love-me vibe. When you're having a bad day or a bad time in life, it's almost impossible. And when you're not getting the love in your life that you need, you can get depressed or anxious or sad and then stuck in your negative feelings, so you give off a gray vibe. You feel stuck in place.

That's why *exercise is so important* when you want self-love. You get up and get moving. The endorphins flood you and your mood instantly improves. Your face gets a healthy flush, and you begin to sweat and detoxify *immediately*. You look like you just got out of bed after a few hours under the sheets with your lover. You're *glowing*. In fact, it's such a palpable glow that I call it the Chi Glow—chi being the life force or the energy inside your body. In my Chi Glow workout, you hold on to glow sticks and do all the exercises in the dark. Talk about *love*!

When you love yourself, you have confidence in your very being. I mean, I know I have a certain look. I like sneakers. I don't wear heels. This is me. If you don't like it, then that's too bad; it doesn't faze me. The last time I went through security at the airport, the TSA agent looked at me with a frown and called me sir. When I corrected her, she felt so bad. Her supervisor then looked at me and said, "Do you go by sir or ma'am?" I replied, "I've never been asked that question, but I go through my life as a woman." And then flashed them a saucy smile, which I could do because I am at ease with myself.

As an aside, do you know how many times a day I get called sir? All day long. Sometimes I think it's a sign that maybe I was meant to be a guy. When I walk around in my life I don't identify as a girl or a boy—I just am. I don't *try* to look like a girl or a boy. I don't have a gender identity; I just look like myself. But it took me most of my life to become comfortable with saying that. After all the years of abusing my body with addictions, I worship it now. I take the best care of it. I love what it is and how it makes me feel.

I only learned how to love myself when I learned how to forgive myself for all the things I messed up and mistakes I made and people I hurt. For instance, I had to stop blaming my dad for leaving when I was little, making me feel abandoned and worthless. In my little girl's mind, I thought he didn't love me, so that meant I wasn't loveable—feelings so deep and buried I didn't even know they were still there. I thought I was doing everything wrong in his eyes, but it was actually just opposite parenting values. My mom was very chill with rules, and my dad was very strict. When I would go to his house for the weekends, I had to switch gears, which made it really hard for me. Rules were not my strong suit. Looking back, I can see how this could have been totally manageable, but that was then and this is now . . . ! But I didn't recognize the depth of this pain until my late twenties, when I started using drugs to mask my pain. Now I've moved way past that. Part of healing is also forgiveness for anyone who's hurt us, and I've forgiven my dad. I love him more than ever. I understand him. And all we can do is move forward toward an even deeper closeness, which feels so unbelievably good.

Another empowering way to self-love is to embrace your body and spirit when they let you down, as they do if you get sick or have a potentially fatal illness. Maria Pargac is one of my longtime students, and she was given a diagnosis of late-stage breast cancer that had spread to some of her lymph nodes. Her oncologist told her it wasn't looking good, that it was likely terminal. During surgery, most of her pectoral muscle was removed, and she was told that due to the trauma, she'd never have muscles there again. She'd be deformed, and weakened, and there was nothing her medical team could do about it.

Maria was determined to get better, and she asked me for help. Before class, I would tell her to visualize her pec muscles coming back, to see herself as whole and strong again. I told her to use her brain to see her body literally pulling the tissue back out and giving her the definition she'd lost during surgery. It worked. Why? Because she took thought and visualizations and backed them up with action, motion, faith, belief, and, most of all, *love*. She manifested her thoughts into reality, physically changing her body with positive affirmations, physical action, and belief in herself. Maria loved herself and she even loved her cancer for forcing her to confront her mortality and focus on the now. All I had to do to help her was acknowledge her hard work, and support her courage and bravery. I am in awe of her courage and drive, and she knows it, which further fueled her determination. Maria is now totally ripped and looks amazing. Her doctors still can't believe it—but they can't argue with the evidence.

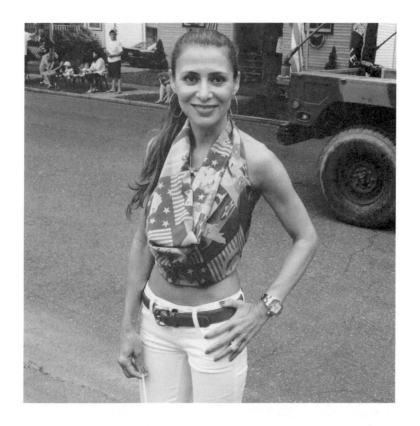

What I knew and what Maria learned is that all exercise is a form of repair. It's all about healthy, deliberate damage to your muscles—creating microtears that, as they heal, make your muscles stronger. Every time you move with intent, you "damage" your body and repair it. That's how you build yourself.

You also want to do something similar to your skin. Did you know that the topmost layer is nothing but dead skin cells linked together in the barrier that protects you from harm?

Well, it is! That's why you need to exfoliate regularly—you need to slough off the dead skin cells with acids (good acids, like those found in fruit or milk) so the fresh, healthy new ones underneath can come to the surface. It's like a controlled burn that sounds scary but does you good.

It's the same thing with your emotions. Slough off the old ones to let the healthy new ones show up, like more love for who you are!

## Visualization for Self-Love

This is an empowering visualization to help you love yourself and give you confidence. Remember, read through this entire visualization at least once before you start. Then try to remember the steps without looking back at the book.

1. Sit in a quiet place and focus on your breathing for a minute. Close your eyes, then picture the words *I LOVE YOU* in your head. Spell out the letters, all eight of them.
2. Make sure you're thinking positively. Make sure you are totally into your breathing, and feeling yourself on a supersensitive level. This is not about anybody else but you. This is your time.
3. Feel your own power, the power you were born with, the power that brought you into this world. Suck your power in and lock it down and hold it so tight. It's *you*. Hold on to you, hug yourself from the inside out. Sometimes there's no one around to give you a hug when you need it, so you hug your-

self. Tighten your abs, and squeeze the tops of your opposite shoulders by crossing your arms. This is a self-hug!

4. Open your mind, open your heart, and feel yourself. Really *feel* yourself. You know that if you can't feel yourself, no one else will ever be able to feel who you are. Feel yourself and love yourself so others can love you, too. This is about a true vibration in your heart.

5. These last few breaths you take are so connected. With your eyes closed, take an above-view look and observe yourself from where you're sitting with your eyes closed. Be proud of your commitment to become connected to who you truly are inside.

6. Open your eyes and come back to the world. Get up and look in the mirror and smile. Because you *are* loveable. And you love yourself. It's kind of weird to say this if you're not used to doing it, I know, but honestly, you won't have to do it that much once you get to the point where you actually do love yourself again. It's that in-between stage when you doubt yourself where you really have to focus on doing it.

As I write this I'm trying to remember the last time I said that. Yep, it's been a while—so I'll be right back! I know that you actually have to do this exercise if you want it to work; just reading about it is not going to help you.

If you're finding yourself struggling with any of the exercises in this book, ask yourself why. Is it ego? Do you not believe in yourself? Do you not believe that positive meditations

# PLAYLIST
## FOR LOVE

Some of my favorite love songs are on this list. Make your own list, too, to reinforce how you feel about your loved ones—and about yourself!

| | |
|---|---|
| Aurora | "Dreaming" |
| Crayon | "Give You Up" |
| Disclosure | "Help Me Lose My Mind" |
| Calvin Harris | "How Deep Is Your Love" |
| Imogen Heap | "Not Now But Soon" |
| Massive Attack | "Protection" |
| Christina Perri | "Thousand Years" |
| The Weekend | "Earned It" |
| Flo Rida ft. Robin Thicke and Verdine Whit | "I Don't Like It, I Love It" |
| RY X | "Only (Kaskade X Lipless Remix)" |

work? This could really be the key to unlocking your emotional blocks. They're all about *you*. Just do them. You have nothing to lose and so much love to gain.

## GOOD, LOVING RELATIONSHIPS ARE LIKE A GOOD JOB—YOU HAVE TO SHOW UP AND DO THE WORK

Relationships are not easy. I burned through so many relationships when I was younger because I'd been taught by the adults in my life that *easy* was the way to behave. Easy might have been the default to allow them to get by when they were struggling, which in retrospect I understand, but it messed up my head and caused me to always look for the way out because the way to stay in was just too hard.

Real love means you have to show up. What I finally learned was that real love takes work.

Because my love is so real, I struggle at times with the work with my girlfriend. I can't say I have always been good at it. We've been a couple for eleven years. Sure, it can be frustrating, but it's so rewarding on every level that I can't imagine not doing the work. My girlfriend has a very high bar for life—and it's not where I was used to living. But I wouldn't be here if it wasn't for her raising the bar on us as a couple. I'd fall back into my old bad habits and patterns. I would not be as busy as I am. She knows that it was in the space between being busy that I'd be tempted to fall backward. It's so easy to get sidetracked. So I keep on doing the work. I have made countless mistakes in our relationship, but we keep going in to make things better all the time. That's where the work pays off.

Staying in love and maintaining a high bar for that love is the most important job you'll ever have. Think of it that way, and you can't possibly say, "Oh, it's a piece of cake." How can such an important job be a breeze? Why *should* it be easy? If you're a parent, you know how hard it is to manage another personality in your life and see the changes in what your children need as they grow—what they need from you and what you need from them.

Raising your kids in this stressful world and launching them into a good place where they are thriving individuals is as tough as it gets. Good parents are my heroes. I see my friends do it. I see my sister do it. I've watched my partner raise three beautiful girls over the last decade. It is the most selfless job anyone could ever take on. She makes it look effortless.

You also have to realize that relationships are always going to evolve over time. The job you loved might become less challenging over the years. The community you loved might have changed as people grew older and moved away or changed their priorities. The little toddler you loved grew up into an independent and feisty teenager with ideas and passions far different from your own. And your partner, whom you vowed to love till death do you part on your wedding day, might not be the same person you fell in love with. He or she might be more loveable—or much, much less.

What made you fall in love and what you thought back then as the most important component in your relationship can shift so completely that you don't even recognize the feelings anymore. Are they still *love?* And are you willing to do the work to keep the relationship thriving? Is your partner? If your relationship is unhappy, are you going to stick it out for the sake of the kids, or is that just an excuse because you'd rather be miserable as a couple than miserable on your own? Are you dreaming about getting out because the grass is always greener and you think if you're not in your current relationship, another one is going to be better?

Only you know the answers to those questions. But there is one common denominator in all thriving, loving relationships, and that's *communication*.

## Good Communication Is a Skill You Can Learn

Good communication is a real issue for me. You know why? Because I have a one-sided conversation for three or four hours a day when I teach. I don't have to listen. I just speak. No one talks back to me, no one challenges me. I'm the boss. And I know my students are really paying attention to me.

You might think because I'm up there teaching and I know what I'm talking about in class that I would automatically be a good listener at home. When I get back to our apartment, I haven't turned off from work mode yet. I'm still used to talking to a rapt audience. When I fall into this trap, what I get in response is a much-deserved "Will you let me finish?" I'm always abashed and apologetic, because I don't even realize I'm going on and on. Factor in my ADHD, and it's a double whammy of having to work extra hard at settling down to have a proper talk. Conversations are always going to be give and take, yin and yang, salt and pepper. It's peanut butter and jelly. Otherwise, one person is giving a monologue and the other person is sitting trapped in the audience.

How do you become better at communicating? At a dinner party once, I asked a very successful journalist—someone who's talked to thousands of people over the course of his career—what makes a good interviewer. "Someone who comes prepared, who asks probing questions, who is genuinely interested in the subject and the person sitting there talking," he told me, "and, most of all, someone who *knows how to listen.*"

"Tell me about it," I said, trying not to roll my eyes. "That's my problem. Not listening hard enough. Sometimes I wish I would get reincarnated as a lap dog. They get unconditional love from their owners, and they don't have to say a word!"

"Well," he said, "I know that if I want to get to the heart of the story, I have to really, *really* listen to what whoever's speaking is saying. I had to teach myself how to do that because when you're reporting, you always have to have the next question in your head, so you have to focus. Sometimes I have to use the interruption technique—which throws people off-base. You're trying to get them to say something they wouldn't have thought of saying, and being interrupted makes them a bit angry or frustrated and then they say something off the prepared script, as it were. It's not like I'm trying to be rude on purpose; it's just to get something interesting out of them." He looked at my face and laughed. "This is a reporter's technique, Stacey," he went on. "Interrupting someone in your personal life is just rudeness, and it won't have the same results. Just ask my wife."

And then he stopped laughing. "You know what I've learned over the course of my career? If I sit down with someone who's not famous and used to being interviewed and stroked all the time, if I sit down with a perfectly nice, average person, and I look them in the eye and say, 'Tell me what happened. Tell me about you. Tell me what's important,' they always will. You know why? Because they're used to no one ever listening to them. To no one thinking their stories are exceptional and worth telling to a stranger who just happens to be a reporter. I see them change, in the span of only a few minutes. They sit up. They remember things they thought they'd forgotten forever. They *are* interesting. Because I've validated them solely by my *active listening*."

"I never thought about it that way," I said.

"It's true," he said. "It's absolutely riveting. And it's a really gratifying part of my job and kind of breaks my heart at the same time. To realize that these people have so much to say and nobody asks them and they don't feel confident enough in themselves to say, 'My opinions are important; I believe in this, somebody please listen to me.' Their kids don't listen, their husband doesn't listen, their boss doesn't listen. They forget how to communicate."

And then you know what happens? When communication goes, love goes. People who aren't listened to and who don't know how to express their needs don't know how to ask for love. They certainly stop loving themselves, and their most needed relationships can break down completely.

Being a better listener will improve all your relationships. I know it's not easy to focus and really pay attention to someone, especially when your mind is going off on tangents or you're tired or hungry or just want to chill. It's also hard when one person is a better communicator than the other, so you can't both stop talking or trying at the same time. If this becomes a problem, one person always has to work even harder at bringing the other person into the conversation. If you both give up, it can be lethal for your relationship.

That's what happened with my partner and me two years ago. We both gave up at the same time even though we promised each other we'd never do that. We got mad at each other and had a horrible fight and we both just went, forget it. *Forget it.* Usually, if we said, "Forget it," I'd say, "No, I'm not going to forget it. We're not going to break up." And we'd clear the air and be fine. But after that horrible fight, it was good-bye. I stormed out. I was devastated. But then after a few months and lots of therapy, we came back together and now our relationship is better than ever.

You know you can't give up if deep in your heart of hearts, you truly love a person. After our brief breakup, I had to work even harder. I had to listen harder. It was worth it, because I'm very lucky to love such an incredible woman with such ferocity, and to have her love me back.

To keep ourselves in touch, she and I text every day. Not two hours go by that we don't touch base. Some might call that codependent, and some might call it love; it doesn't matter to me because communication keeps our relationship healthy. It works for us, and I'm sure you can find something that works for you. I never stop thinking about sweet and silly little things that might make her happy, and vice versa. If we both had super-busy workdays and not much time for talking or texting, on the way home I might stop and get a card, or buy her an item for the house that she mentioned she wanted. (One of these items was an electric sesame seed distributor—definitely not something that would ever be on my radar!) It's not that she needed an electric sesame seed distributor, or any other object—it's that I listened to her, remembered what she said, and acted on it.

Or, if I need space, I'll say, "I'm going to turn off my phone for a few hours while I do some writing or have to take a twenty-minute nap." Then I text when I'm back. You don't have to hide or lie that you're going to be somewhere that you're not if you need space. Everyone needs space, breathing room, time on their own. I have a hard time asking for it. I get super bitey and then I know I just need to get out and go do something for myself. The second you just take ownership of your time, you'll feel better.

Just tell your partner what you're doing! And listen to your partner when they say they need space, too.

The more skilled you are at listening, the better you will become at seeing people for who they really are. You will be more judicious in who you give your heart to. And you *will* attract all kinds of love into your life.

## Never Go to Sleep Angry

One rule we have in our house is that no one can ever go to bed angry.

If you do, you can kiss a good night's sleep good-bye. You'll have crazy weird dreams, because your brain can't chill and settle down. You'll start the next day off on the wrong foot.

You need to get whatever is plaguing you out of your brain and body, somehow, before you go to sleep. Let your partner know you want to try to fix things and have some good pillow talk. And great sex allows you to regroup (as long as it's *connected* sex, that is—disconnected sex or withholding sex is guaranteed to exacerbate any anger, right?). It makes you feel pretty damn good, too!

Holding on to anger or grudges not only prevents any kind of open and helpful communication, it destroys relationships before you can say "WTF." Grudges are toxic. They make you angry and then you radiate this rage that pushes people away. I am the worst at this, actually. I have classically hung on to stuff without talking about it, and it piles up on my heart and then I explode. I have learned to really talk about the way I feel *before* it annoys me.

You need to communicate with the person you're mad at, but sometimes, for whatever reason, you haven't been able to get your message across. Sometimes it's because the person is no longer available (through distance, or even death), or sometimes it's because, if you're honest, you want to remain the victim instead of dealing with the situation.

---

SG TRUTH   **I am really bad at talking about what bothers me. I actually have to make sure I am communicating on a daily basis, and that takes a *lot* of work.**

---

My suggestion is to have the grudge-busting conversation with this person anyway. Either in your head, or by talking out loud to an empty room, or by writing a letter or e-mail and *not* saving it in your drafts before you send it. Send it only to *yourself.* Fine-tune it as much as you like. The mere act of saying or writing down what you need to say is a huge help at getting the grudge out of your system, even if you have been very wronged.

Then, if you've written anything down on paper, take a match to it and burn it up. You're burning away the anger, and you are moving on to a more loving place. Then you can present yourself nicely to the parties involved. (Obviously, burning a letter can be very dangerous, so don't do it in the house unless it is a very small piece of paper being burned at the bottom of a very deep sink. If you have a fireplace, you're in luck—otherwise, take it outside to a safe place.)

## Good Communication Fosters Intimacy

I never liked talking about the past. It was too painful. My therapist helped me work out that as long as I held back, I could never cross that wondrous line that takes a relationship from just okay to the best it can be. That's what I call the Intimacy Line.

Intimacy is key to love in a relationship. Intimacy is trust. Intimacy fosters communication because this trust makes you unafraid to share your deepest needs and issues without fear of being judged. Knowing that your partner or your friends have your back no matter what is the best feeling in the world.

What I wonder and worry about is how social media is changing the way people's brains work, especially as it creates fake intimacy. You can develop relationships with people that you think are deep and meaningful but that are wholly virtual. I'm not saying these relationships can't be amazing, but they're still digital. And that makes them nonintimate. (It can also make them devastatingly disappointing, if you spend days or weeks or even months involved in a virtual relationship.) The only way you can have true intimacy is with a real person in a real place, looking at each other in real time and having real reactions. In other words, you need to be an analog lover.

I had a friend who went on an app called Second Life, a popular online community that allows you to create the "life" you want. You can create your house, your apartment, your avatar, your family, even your pets. You talk to other Second Lifers as your avatar. My friend got so hooked on it that he started spending up to twelve hours a day on it. His work suffered. And his marriage suffered more. It ended. It wasn't just the time he spent on the game—it was how his avatar was a wholly different person, not one his wife would have ever recognized, but it served as a distraction for him and the pain he was going through in his real life. The game was an escape from his inability to communicate his true feelings. For years this distraction went on and just prolonged his being able to find genuine joy.

Some couples—not anyone I know well, but a lot I know *of*— are merely two people who are together but not in a deep way, and they don't really like talking at the end of the day. They might not have the kind of intimacy I have with my partner, but it could still be a great surface-level relationship. A lot of people prefer to function on the surface because they're unable or unwilling to go deeper. They might shun therapy. They might be happy with things the way they are. If so, and if they're *truly* happy, then fine. Whatever floats your boat.

The key issue is whether or not these couples are *truly* happy. I don't see how some people can be without intimacy, but that's me. I'm not sayin' it has to be rockin' every night of your life with your partner, but you should feel intimate toward them often! I wasn't truly happy in many of my prior relationships because I wasn't able to be truly intimate. Often, I walked away; other times, my then girlfriend did. All of us have made errors in judgment about people.

## Exercise and Your Sex Life

There are three wonderful ways exercise improves your sex life.

Let's call on the American Council on Exercise for the first one, as they state that being physically active can be "a natural Viagra boost."

This is thanks to endorphins. These are the compounds produced by the hypothalamus and the pituitary gland in your brain; they're released during exercise, excitement, pain—and orgasm. Endorphins give you what's called a "runner's high," even though you don't have to be running to feel that rush. You just have to be *moving*. In bed or out!

The second way is that exercise strengthens and conditions your body for the intensely physical act of lovemaking. A strong cardiovascular system will give you the stamina so you can go and go and go. Firm muscles and flexibility will allow you to experiment and enjoy trying different positions. Exercise also dilates your arteries and improves blood flow. Men need this to sustain their erections; women need this to help arouse their genitals.

Being fit through exercise is especially important for men worried about their sexual performance. Numerous studies at the Harvard School of Public Health and elsewhere have also shown how exercise especially helps men improve their production of dihydrotestosterone, or DHT, a potent form of testosterone. According to Dr. Harry Fisch, a New York City–based urologist and author of *The New Naked: The Ultimate Sex Educa-*

*tion for Grown-Ups,* "A man's body must have adequate testosterone levels to build muscle mass, so someone who is fit and muscled is likely to have normal or high levels of testosterone."

The higher the testosterone, as you likely know, the higher the sex drive and the less likelihood of erectile dysfunction or impotence. The heavier a man's weight, though, especially if he tends to gain it in his midsection, the *lower* his testosterone levels. He won't just have performance problems—his libido will falter as well.

The third way exercise improves your sex life has to do with body image. Obviously, you don't need a "great" or unrealistically "perfect" porn body for sex. But one of the biggest reasons women don't like to have sex is because they don't feel good about their bodies. They think they're fat when they're not. They're worried about their jiggly bits. They don't want to be shamed and found wanting when they're naked and vulnerable.

Exercise can undo all that self-shaming that I wish would disappear for good. It gives you confidence. It makes you feel good in every possible way. It makes you appreciate how your body works and what it's capable of doing. I see body confidence growing in my students the more they work out. This isn't about weight loss, but about that *confidence.* They literally stand taller. They carry themselves completely differently, and it's not just because their core is stronger and their glutes firmer. It's because they finally feel happy about their physicality—and for you, this will translate to feeling happy about yourself whether the lights are on or off.

Think about this in the context of all the ads you see that are hyping exercise-related activities and merchandise. How do the models look? Well, of course they look buff—but they also have the glow. They positively radiate healthy, sexual energy. It's not just because they're selling something—it's because working out makes you look and feel sexy! Forget sex appeal—I call it *flex* appeal.

And you don't have to be young like most of the fitness models to have flex appeal. It's a state of mind *and* muscles. (Jack LaLanne sure had it up until the end!) Kelly Ripa once jokingly quoted me on her show when she said, "For women over forty, the universe is trying to suck the back of your arms into the center of the earth." Yes, gravity is a bitch, but flex appeal can counteract its effects—if you let it. Kelly isn't exactly a twenty-year-old; she was born in 1970 but looks better now than she ever has. She is fully at ease in her body and with who she is.

Some of my friends and students aren't as body-confident as I am (or as Kelly is!), and sometimes they ask what they should do when they're feeling vulnerable about their body and have a new lover. I suggest that they get some fabulous lingerie and leave the top on. To light a lot of candles and make their bedroom atmospherically sexy. But you know what? You are almost always going to be judging yourself more harshly than your lover is. The only kind of lover you want to have is one who loves your body for what it is.

Radiating sexual confidence is what makes you attractive. You will always have the best sex when you can let your inhibitions go and get out of your own way. That is extremely difficult to do if you are worried about someone seeing your cellulite or scars or a little pooch in your belly and judging you. (As for scars, to me they're like badges of honor, markers in your story, and a reminder of experiences only you have had. They're like dropping a pin on a place in time—that's all a scar is.) You have to get out of that cycle of thinking your sexual partner is somehow rating you on their own mental scale of perceived worthiness. And if you're with someone who's judging you on any aspect of your body, it's the wrong person. The quickest way to ruin a relationship is to be critical of sexual performance or any physical characteristics.

Although some of my students often pull me aside to whisper and confide in me about why they've got that special glow—the one that comes not just from regular exercise, but from a thriving and pleasurable sex life, it takes time for others to reach that point. One of the most gratifying things for me to see—and this has happened countless times in my thirty years of teaching, not just with my students but with my friends and acquaintances—is when someone who has retreated into themselves and basically given up on sex and dating then finds the will to get moving. They start working out regularly and effectively. They lose weight, get stronger, feel better in every possible way, and rediscovers the marvel of their body. They start dating again and they start having sex again, and they are much happier.

My friend Noa is someone who didn't date for more than a decade; he thought no one would find him attractive because

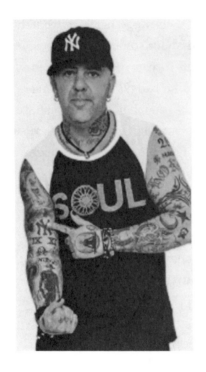

*he* didn't find himself attractive due to his weight. We became good friends when we both were living in Los Angeles. He actually asked me, leaning out the window of his car one night at midnight, to help him change his life. I looked at him and said, "Let's do it."

We trained together for about a year, and then I moved to New York. Several years later, he went out to buy some underwear at H&M, and he happened to walk past the opening day of the West Hollywood branch of SoulCycle. He decided to give it a try and signed up for a few classes. Although he had once been fit, he then weighed more than three hundred pounds. He was deeply ashamed of his body, and his doctor had basically told him that he could drop dead of a heart attack at any moment. (For him to even think about leaving the house to go underwear shopping was a big deal.) When he saw the new SoulCycle, he thought he might as well die trying, and once he got on that bike, what kept him going during that first class was, he told me later, remembering how I used to tell him, during our training sessions, "If you are here, you *are* an athlete! The hard work is getting yourself here, today."

Since that day, not only did Noa lose more than one hundred pounds, but he was freed, as he put it, "from the bondage of being my former self." Even more amazing, he was encouraged to train to become a SoulCycle instructor—and he now teaches at several of the NYC studios. He might call himself an "old dog that did actually learn some new tricks," but we both agree that his transformation came about because he found his purpose.

And he also realized that women found him extremely attractive. He told me that what he'd thought was a cliché—that it's written all over your body when you have physical and emotional confidence—was actually true, and he was living proof.

So . . . what are you waiting for?

While I always want people to make the decision to get exercising because it's so good for them, sometimes it takes an outside event to spur their motivation. I've lost track of how many students have told me over the years that their "breakup workout" ended up not only improving their health but healing their broken hearts. This is what happened to Alicia. When her husband, Ben, left her for another woman, she was devastated. Not only because she'd been in love with him, but because his new girlfriend was in phenomenal physical shape, and Ben made sure Alicia knew it. (Don't get me started on this guy; at least she's well rid of him!)

"He used to love my body," Alicia told me. "Sure, I could

have worked out a bit more, but I was strong and healthy and not overweight at all. He loved to caress what he called my sweet, soft arms. And then he started complaining about my 'out-of-shape arms,' and before long he was ragging on me about my entire body."

Ben was about as shallow as it gets, not just for dumping Alicia in the way he did, but for criticizing her body and no longer appreciating who she was on the inside, where it really counts. So what does this have to do with a better sex life?

Well, let's just say that Alicia took that hurt right to the gym, where she worked out with more intensity than she had before. She didn't care about Ben anymore—she now cared about *herself*. Over time, I noticed that Alicia was looking better and better. But I'm not just talking about more muscle tone. Her attitude had shifted.

One day, after class, we started chatting, and she told me she felt like a new woman. When I asked her what she meant, she said, "Well, after I got divorced, I never thought I'd feel good about anything again. When I started dating again, I have to admit I was a bit shocked to find how sexy I felt. I have more sexual confidence now that I've never had before."

Being in shape is not about sex. Being in shape is all about feeling sexy . . . about feeling so great about yourself that the thought of being seen naked and getting intimate and having sex doesn't inspire panic or fear. And that's the best kind of confidence a person can have.

## Moving Meditation for Intimacy

This is a small and subtle thing to do, but it works as a connection to your intimate self. You can do it anytime and any place you feel the need for an intimate connection. It pulls together all your senses and opens you up to loving the touch of your skin and your innate sensuality. When you are done, you will be ready to embrace any kind of intimate encounter.

1. Take your thumb and touch your index fingertip, gently, barely feeling your skin, and make tiny soft circles in a clockwise direction. Don't focus on counting or doing this for a specific amount of time. Keep making the circles until you feel ready to move on.
2. Repeat with your middle finger, then your ring finger, and then your pinkie.
3. Open your hand wide and then close it into a loose fist. Hold that moment in your hand.
4. Repeat with your other hand.

Now your senses are alert. . . . Stay in touch with this sensation. It is the total secret to staying physically "in touch" with your sensuality.

## PUSHING PAST SHAME

When it comes to training your heart and opening it up to love, shame is a big one. Getting found out. Being exposed. Feeling like a failure. I mean, we all have things we are ashamed of, that we'd rather crawl into a cave than admit to, so we remain stuck in the layers and moments that once shamed us—even, of course, if we were totally blameless when the shaming happened. If, for example, you grow up in a house where you're constantly criticized and not allowed to express your feelings, if you're told *no, no, no, why, why, why* all the time, you internalize that terrible feeling that you're not good enough and never will be. The worst feelings of inadequacy are that you're not deserving of love and happiness and purpose. You're ashamed to think you deserve the best. When this happens, you can unwittingly be holding yourself back for fear of failing and repeating the shame, especially when you're trying to get motivated.

One of the reasons people are afraid to ask for help is due to shame. Especially if you said you were going to do something important (look for a new job, lose weight, exercise more) and for whatever reasons that something doesn't happen. You're ashamed that you weren't able to succeed. I totally get it, because shame keeps addicts addicted. If you think you're not worthy because you're doing something that is bad/illegal/toxic, then it's easier to stay stuck in the shame and guilt than to go to rehab and kick the habit. It took me many, many years to own up to my shame. And believe me, I am not perfect. There's still a lot of work I have to do on myself, so you are not alone, my friend!

I was only able to become as successful when I started to

deal with my layers of shame and to acknowledge that this would be an ongoing thing for me. It's one of those issues I will always have to deal with, even if much of the shame is usually tucked away. For example, I can speak as a former drug addict, but it's harder for me to identify as an alcoholic due to shame. I come from a long line of alcoholics, and even if most of my friends growing up did, too, it was still something we rarely talked about, and if we did, we did it laughing.

Doesn't that self-identification stuff sound a bit nutty? But it's because I would do drugs before I would do alcohol. Usually it's the other way around. My buzz of choice came from drugs, not drinks. Drugs were always my go-to for self-medication. I don't like the feeling of being drunk, so it's hard for me to identify as an alcoholic, but apparently as part of sobriety you're supposed to say that you're an alcoholic if you're a drug addict. I think maybe I have to tell myself I *am* an alcoholic. If I don't, then I run the risk of thinking about having a drink.

Instead, I've convinced myself that I'm allergic to alcohol. I mean, I'm not *physically* allergic to alcohol, but I am *emotionally*. Like many drinkers, when I drink I become a different person. It usually took about three and a half drinks for me to morph from being funny, happy, loving, and great company into a total asshole. So that means I'm allergic to drinking. I tell myself that so my brain's response to someone drinking isn't to say, "Oh, I wish I could have a drink," but "If I have a drink, I'm going to feel awful because I'm allergic. Don't be a fool. It's toxic. If you have a drink, you're going to have a bad reaction and you're going to be sorry. You're going to feel like complete crap with your stupid hangover. Also, you will lose *everything* you have ever worked for in your life if you drink. None of that is worth it, so have a Pellegrino and go enjoy yourself."

The greatest thing about saying *no* to drugs and alcohol is the empowerment and self-control it gives you. What you have to steer clear of, however, are the triggers that can bring you right back into that behavior. Believe it or not, sometimes it's not even the alcohol or the drug that triggers you—it can be a person who makes you feel the same way. Be super sensitive to your surroundings, and don't let anyone take you down the rabbit hole toward disrespectful behavior, because it can happen.

Still, shame will rear its unwanted little face when I least expect it, such as in a topic of seemingly benign conversation at a dinner party. Maybe I'll be at a dinner with a few people who don't know me well, and they'll be asking what I want to drink, and I'll say, "I'll have a Pellegrino, please." A savvy host or hostess would then get that drink for me without comment, but some hosts or hostesses are not so savvy. They'll push it because everyone is drinking (and maybe they're actually alcoholics who can't own up to and hate to be around nondrinkers), and then it gets into why can't I have a drink. *That* is the moment where the shame hits. When a stranger says, "Oh,

SG, circa 1996

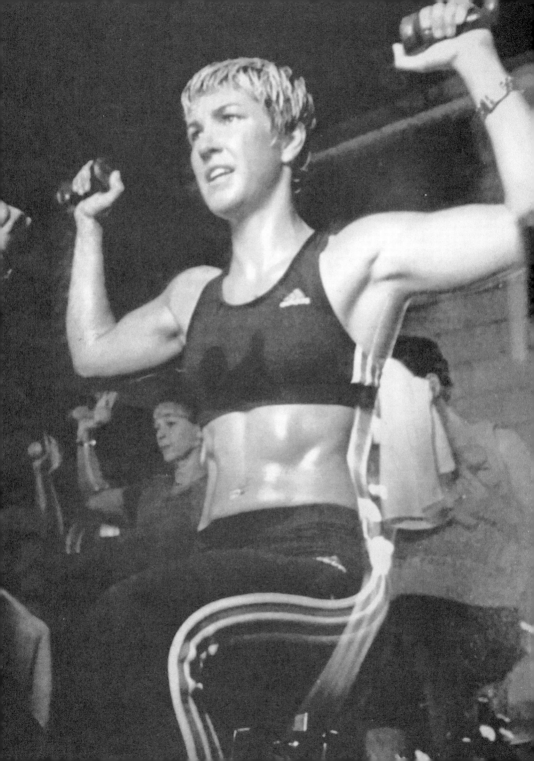

come on, Stacey, just have one." Whenever I hear that, it's like a vise has gotten a stranglehold on my heart for a brief second. It's not exactly *painful,* but it's awfully uncomfortable. It's pure shame. And it's still there, even after all my years of sobriety. It gets easier with every passing year, though, so that's good!

The shame of having been an addict for so long used to make me really fearful in some social situations, because I've had so many years of sobriety, and Sober Stacey is who I identify with now. The smart and reliable Stacey who is a fitness instructor who's never taught a class in New York City with a wicked hangover. My identity used to be Crazy Stacey, Hurricane Stacey, Stacey the life of the party, Stacey the addict who had tons of friends and knew everyone. Stacey who could party and still show up to classes the next day. Stacey who was the woman to call whenever you wanted to have fun. . . .

So my shame is not fear-based anymore—the fear stemming from people finding out I was an addict and judging me accordingly—but it's still that piece of me and my life that I wish I didn't have to have anymore. I mean, it's part of who I am, but I prefer to identify with people now who feel and behave like I do—with sober intent, with passion, and with a hard look inside themselves.

It's *hard* not to have a crutch like drinking or drugging, especially in the fitness industry where, surprisingly enough, not that many instructors are fully clean and sober. When you grew up drinking and drugging, it's hard not to drink or smoke pot or have that line of cocaine at a party. Society might pretend otherwise, but there's tons of drugs everywhere, and for most people, it's really hard to say no to a glass of wine or other alcohol.

One of my most deeply shameful moments was during the wrap party for a big event. The hostess was incredibly generous and loved nothing more than giving back, and at this party everyone was so happy and celebrating. She was pouring shots of tequila, and I'm standing there, and she turned to me to give me a shot.

What flashed into my head at that moment was, *Damn it all, Stacey, you want to be a part; you want to be in the club.* If I had chosen a night when it would have been a perfect time to fall off the wagon, it would have been that night.

And then something else flashed into my head—the right answer. So, instead, I said no.

She didn't know I had been an addict and was "allergic" to alcohol, and it was certainly not the time or place to tell her, so she, in her generous way, kept trying to hand me the shot. To avoid hurting her feelings, I took it and quickly gave it to someone else. As the party went on, people were actually shocked when they realized I wasn't drinking. I was having a blast anyway, dancing all over the room all night. (I even ended up dancing on top of the speakers!) It was a fabulous party with fabulous people, and I knew I didn't need alcohol to make it better. I truly did not need a shot to celebrate our accomplishments. I can celebrate standing right next to you while you do your thing.

The point is, in our society, alcohol is used for celebrations the way sugar is. After all, what's a birthday party without a cake? But even though I had a brilliant time at the party, the shame was still nagging at me. I couldn't tell the hostess the truth that night and buzzkill the moment. Because shame is your deepest secrets about stuff you did that you think makes you a bad person—a person unworthy of love.

## Truth Telling Is the Shame Killer

How do you push past the shame, allowing you to feel worthy of the love you deserve?

I learned from my therapist that shame is just you being found out, and when you walk through your life with the shame you become an imposter. To yourself and to everyone else.

I know all my addiction issues. I understand exactly what each drug made me feel and why I did everything I did. I've come to terms with it. I self-medicated with crystal meth because I had ADHD chronic-fatigue and the meth made me feel awake. I was suffering from depression because my brother had died. I was so sad I started doing a lot of Ecstasy because that was making me happy. My emotions at the time, in response to these drugs, were still authentic.

All the drugs made my real senses come straight to the edge of my skin. I wasn't masking any feelings; if anything, I was bringing them up. When you do Ecstasy and meth you talk about anything and everything. I was already a talker, of course, but *not* about my *feelings*. I'm actually very shy. I learned from a young age that my family story was something shameful to my peers. I would try to hide the fact that my parents were divorced and I was from a single-parent home. And then when I knew I was gay, I knew that was a secret I had to keep.

As a result, as you know already, I grew up in lies. I wasn't ashamed of being gay, but I knew that *others* saw it as shameful, and I had to lie to protect myself from the cruelty of their homophobia. Since I grew up having to lie about my identity, about being straight or gay, "Oh yeah, this is my boyfriend," "Oh yeah, these are my parents," sometimes it's still my knee-jerk reaction—to tell a white lie. It's very, *very* hard to unwind that. Why should I feel ashamed about the lies I had to tell in self-preservation when I was younger?

But I still do. Because being a liar was *easy*. I would never have been able to admit that without having been in therapy for the last decade. Do you know how brave it is to tell people that you were a liar? Do you know how hard it is to admit you were a drug addict? How much more open and exposed can you get? I had to push past the shame. I could do it only because I fell in love with a person who believed in me, and loved me the way I was. Having her in my life made me realize that the only way our relationship could work was if I was honest about everything that happened to me. So I did. I killed my shame with the truth.

Telling the unvarnished truth is like peeling the layers

back on the onion of vulnerability. It's almost impossible to get through your entire day without telling a lie. You know you have to come up with those little white lies because you don't want to tell your friend that, yes, her little black dress actually does make her look fat, or tell your boss that he's an incompetent hack with bad breath. You don't want to hurt your friend's feelings and you don't want to get fired. In other words, there's a difference between the little lies you tell to survive, and the bigger lies you tell yourself.

You also need to find something that pushes you out of being stuck in the holding-on-to-shame pattern. If you keep telling yourself that you're bad and unworthy, if you think you can't undo what was done, then you have to take action. Either by unburdening yourself to someone trustworthy who can help (as my therapist helped me), or by creating a new reality for yourself.

Confidence is key. If you're really good at something—and everybody is, whether it's running a multibillion-dollar company or having a really lovely potted garden on your porch— you can push past shame, too. You don't have to think you're unworthy anymore. And your confidence about yourself begets more confidence, which makes you exude happiness, which brings love to you. The trick is to keep your momentum, and that, as you know, means *moving* and staying in shape!

Instead of the shame driving you, go back to your MAP. Make a Plan. Do it now. Instead of telling yourself you're a failure, say, "I have a plan. I have a MAP. I am going to be like a toddler learning to walk. That toddler falls down and gets up again and falls down and gets up again. If toddlers stopped trying the first time they fell down, they'd still be crawling. They don't criticize themselves or think they're no good at walking. They get up. They know they can do it. They're confident that they're going to figure it out and succeed. And I will, too."

If those toddlers fall too many times and get tired and frustrated, what do they do? They cry. They're preverbal, and the only way they can communicate and ask for help is with their tears. There's no shame in crying. Sometimes as human beings we don't give love and attention until someone's crying, and then we soften up because we see the upset. Besides, sometimes a good cry can be incredibly cathartic, to help clear out the mental garbage and jargon that's bringing you down.

## The Rule of Nine Is a Shame Killer, Too

If you're still having trouble with your shame issues, try this: For every one bad thing you did, or do, I believe that you can do nine good things to get rid of that one bad thing. That's how you match up your karma. If you fuck something up, you've got to make nine people's lives better for that one fuck-up.

The Rule of Nine doesn't have to be about large things. It can be as small as buying a sandwich for the homeless person in your neighborhood or as big as helping your friend pack up her house when she has to downsize because she lost her job.

It can be telling your friend who borrowed fifty dollars from you that they don't ever have to pay it back—it's a gift. It's about helping someone move on a Sunday when it's your only day off. It's about driving an hour to sit shivah for your friend's grandmother whom you never met. It's about letting someone stay with you when they're going through a hard time and need a place to crash for a while. Doing these good deeds will fill your heart up. Do as many as you can.

## FLIP THE NEGATIVE

When you're training your heart and opening it up to love, it helps to process your feelings of hurt and pain by seeing the good components of whatever it is that's hurting you. In other words, flip the negative and make it positive.

Tell yourself this (and *believe* it): Every emotion is temporary, and every time you blink is a chance to change your attitude. You're now going to be all about exuding self-love.

For example, if there is a painful memory (an argument, a deep hurt, the loss of a loved one), hold on to all the best moments between you and that person. Don't be afraid to create a dialogue in your head with that person. Have the same conversation you would have had if they were sitting in the same room with you. It's comforting to know they might be listening to you. It's just faith. Have it—it works.

Or another: If you discover that your partner is cheating and decides to leave your marriage . . . deal with the anger. Adjust to the changes. Then see the great moments (your wedding day, the first house, the amazing children) and hang on to those. Delete the bad; it only drags down your energies. Admit you understand, on a profound level, deep down, why your partner left, even if the future is scary.

Or another: Loss of a job only means your next opportunity is waiting for you around the corner, but you have to put on your discovery hat and be an adventurer to go seek it out. Don't wait for it to fall in your lap—you have to manifest it. Which is why the group dynamic is so special. You will network into so many amazing circles of life, and by getting to know the people around you, you put out the things you need, and the universe will take care of the rest. This is not hokey, by the way. This is you setting an intention, using your life experiences to meet up with the right opportunities, and acting upon it.

Emotional presence in your life is the quintessential ingredient to a healthy mind and body. You *have* to stay connected to your true feelings in order to train your heart.

Believe me, I know how hard this can be. Especially if you are a drinker, or a pill popper. I can't drink or take pills for *anything* anymore, which means I basically go through life feeling every single emotion, every uncomfortable moment, every thrilling moment, 100 percent present in my mind and body. I never thought I could survive without being numbed.

But once I was sober I discovered I like it this way. It's the real me, shame and all. It's also the most powerful feeling, waking up in my body every day!

Know your pitfalls and walk through them, not around them. That's flipping the negative. Walking around them keeps you in them; walking through them allows you to feel the bottom, and know that you don't belong there.

If, for instance, your pitfall is drinking, walking through it means telling yourself you can't drink like that because you experienced the feeling of doing it already. You can't walk down it again. I use these metaphors to replace that fear with confidence—to acknowledge the real feelings of the real you.

## PUT YOURSELF IN THE MIX AND CHANGE IT UP

When I was a DJ, my friend Brett called me DJ Miss Mix-y. Because I was always mixing. Not just music for the dance floor—I was always mixing people together, inviting different people to different events. I wanted all my friends to blend and mix it up. I had straight friends, I had gay friends, I had models, actors, schoolteachers, construction workers, lawyers, and doctors in my life. I especially loved taking my straight friends with straight jobs to gay parties. They always had a blast. I would say to them, "Just go out there and put yourself in the mix."

Putting yourself into the mix isn't just about music. It's about doing whatever you need to do to shake up your life. This will bring new people into your orbit. It will also bring new opportunities and new confidence. And more love into your heart.

Start mixing it up by doing something as simple as changing how you get to work, or where you go for lunch. This is especially important when you're feeling stuck. A new routine is a must when your old routine isn't doing it for you anymore. If you go to lunch at noon every day, at the same place show up at eleven forty-five instead, somewhere else. Sure, there is comfort in being a regular somewhere, but there's also comfort in knowing you're capable of putting yourself in the mix.

Get out your bucket list and start doing something about it. Maybe go on a trip with a group once in a while (even if it's just a day-trip to a park or to take a hike in the woods), sign up for a surf camp in Costa Rica, or go on a cruise by yourself!

Putting yourself in the mix is, on a more profound level, about taking risks. You've got to go for it (whatever it is) to get it. Well, I think we all know that falling in love is the biggest risk you'll take.

That's why I love my girlfriend so much. She's such a lover of life. She might be a hard-ass, but I love her even more for that. She runs a tight ship, but that's why we've worked through our problems and are now two years past our ten-year anniversary and happier than ever. Her rules are inviolable, and thank goodness for that. Remember, I was taught to go for easy, which got me precisely nowhere—so it can get uncomfortable for me when my buttons get pushed. But it keeps me on my toes. It keeps our relationship fresh. If it were too easy and plugged in to my comfort zone, I'd soon be bored out of my brain. I'd be drinking and using again because I'd have too much time on my hands, looking for fun and something to keep me occupied. Instead of doing the hard, challenging work of training my heart.

What I've also learned is that you can't *not* love in fear of rejection or losing it. Part of love is losing it. I have had my heart broken so many times, but that didn't stop me from pursuing future relationships. I don't *not* love because of my past. Right now, the thought of me *not* being with my girlfriend is so devastating I don't even think about it. But if that ever did happen, for whatever reason, I'd have to deal with it then. Projecting wild fears into the future is a dumb kind of risk. You risk projecting hypothetical ideas into the now. For what purpose?

Stick to your MAP. Evaluate the pros and cons of the risks you're considering. Then . . . go for it!

## THE ALTRUISM OF LOVE

Want to know how to have a bad relationship? It's simple. It's not seeing someone for who they are, and deciding that you can "fix" and mold the person into who you want them to be.

Except people can't be "fixed" if they don't want to be fixed. They'll change only when they're ready (and many never will be).

You can't make someone love you the way you want them to love you. They either do or they don't. If you fall into this trap, you can't blame the other person. This can turn into a vicious cycle and be a relationship-killer because you might just want your partner to be the best they can be so you can grow together, side by side. But if your partner doesn't want your help, or can't accept it, you've got a problem. I am always willing to try harder, but that's usually after my mild tantrum of "I can't do this any better. . . ." Then I catch myself and say, "I'll try harder."

In other words, there is an enormous difference between self-sacrifice and altruism.

Self-sacrifice can veer precipitously from love and admiration to martyrdom and accusations. Altruism, on the other hand, is what you want to strive for in a relationship.

My trusty dictionary defines altruism as "the belief in or practice of disinterested and selfless concern for the well-being of others." Teachers, doctors, and social workers are altruistic by profession. Trainers and healers are, too. That is really who I am, because I love helping people feel better and look better and do better. That's my calling. It's my purpose. On that long-ago day in church, Pastor Bayless's mom told me I was chosen to speak. I didn't quite get it at the time, but I've gotten it now. I found the channel for my message—which is *exercise*. To get moving and to keep moving.

An altruistic relationship is based on mutual respect, honesty, and communication. *Both* of you are "practicing selfless concern for the well-being" of each other, at the *same* time. It's working toward the same goals.

What you should both try to do is *out love* each other. Try to love harder. If you're both on the same altruistic page, you'll never go wrong.

If you have a relationship like that now, I salute you. If not, you *can* have it. He or she is out there for you. Focus on your visualizations. Get busy. Throw your positive vibes out into the universe. Accept your faults. Get help pushing past the dark emotions and memories that might be holding you back. Love yourself a whole lot more, and you're going to *shine* so bright you will be the beacon that leads love toward you.

## Visualization for Love

This is a very powerful visualization for bringing love and magic into your life.

1. Sit in a comfortable position in a dark room. Close your eyes.
2. Picture yourself as energy, as if you were your own Hubble telescope peering out at all the stars in the universe. We are all energies. We are all force fields walking through this universe.

3. Keep imagining what your energy looks like, and try to put your hands on it. When you capture it, it's like that magic moment when your children collect fireflies at night. When your children stare at the jar full of life and love.

4. Imagine your energy filling up an enormous and special jar of life and love. Feel it in your heart. Let it heal you. Let this light of love heal everybody you touch. This is how you change the world and this is how you find love. Feel your body glow. Get brighter and brighter. Brighter and brighter.

5. Now from the inside out, give yourself a huge hug by grabbing your hips right hand to left hip and left hip to right hand, and then flex your abs. Send the love vibration through your body, and watch how differently you feel when you open your eyes. Do it now!

"All athletes know they have to fuel the machine properly."

# SEVEN

## EAT

No matter how hard you work out, if you don't eat right, you won't get results. The truth is that most of what you look like is based on what you put in your mouth.

In large part because I always ate well, I was able to function and continue to work in the fitness industry during my years as an addict. All athletes know they have to fuel the machine properly, whether they're deep in training or not, or they'll never come out on top. You know that I believe we're all capable of being athletes, but don't think that because you're not a *professional* athlete, you can eat what you want now and pay for it later. Sure you can—you pay for it later by being overweight, unhealthy, or dead!

What I've learned from my thousands of students over the years is that there are three reasons, and three reasons alone, why they want to lose weight *now:*

- Fear ("I'm afraid of getting sick/getting ignored/getting stuck/not looking good for an event or job.")
- Revenge ("I'll show that loser who just dumped me what he's/she's missing!")
- Love ("I want to look fab for my love.")

What's missing from this list, of course, is that everyone should want to be at a normal weight—note that this doesn't mean the bone-thin size o so beloved of the misguided fashion industry and media—in order to be as *healthy* as possible for as long as possible. Until you love yourself enough to make good eating habits part of your lifetime routine, you're just going to make it harder to attain and maintain results.

This is why you need to acknowledge your intentions about making a realistic eating plan a regular part of your life. Use the suggestions in this chapter to help you identify and deal with the emotional issues about your weight that might be holding you back.

## EATING FOR INTENT

What do you reach for when you want an extra boost of energy before a workout or an intense meeting at work? What is your comfort food when you're blue? Is there one particular food that trips you up every time you vow to change how you eat?

Food affects moods. (Look at the words *food* and *mood*—they are literally one letter apart.) Not just from blood sugar spikes, but because every food contains nutrients with specific properties. I also believe that because food has such a profound effect on moods, it's one of the reasons why diets don't work. If you're in a bad mood, eating something calming can help bring you back to chill. If you're too tired to go to the gym, drinking something fresh and energizing can give you that pop you need. Being super restrictive about what you eat (and staring at that *number* on the scale) is a recipe for failure. Instead, stock your shelves with all kinds of nutritious foods that do for your body what visualizations and Moving Meditations do for your spirit. You already did your kitchen declutter, right? (If not, turn back to page 140!) Those nice empty shelves are practically begging for healthy and delicious items to be placed on them.

I don't believe in diets. We all know they don't work. Instead of *diet*s, I believe in *live*-its. I believe in setting your intentions about how and what and why you want to eat what you do, and how you want to feel. There are always choices. Be deliberate in them and you will automatically feel better and lose weight.

# THE BEST ENERGIZING FOODS FOR EVERYDAY LIFE

My holistic nutrition consultant and wellness curator Meredith and I compiled these lists of the best foods for your needs. These foods are nutrient dense and full of vital minerals and vitamins that help build healthy cells, strong bodies, and powerful minds. Fresh is always best. Frozen is okay. (Canned foods are not something I recommend, because the linings of some cans contain an endocrine-disrupting chemical called BPA that can leach into the food.)

- Bee pollen. It's loaded with protein, vitamins, and folic acid. The best is locally sourced. One teaspoon usually does the trick, but avoid it, of course, if you're allergic to bees!
- Beets, raw, cooked, or as fresh juice. I love beets! They're super detoxifying and sweet enough to curb cravings.
- Cacao. This dark chocolate is super dense in magnesium, which you need for muscle and cognitive functioning as well as heart health.
- Coconut milk. It's loaded with healthy, naturally occurring saturated fat containing 50 percent lauric acid, a medium-chain fatty acid that is quickly assimilated for an energy boost. Fresh coconut milk is far superior to canned.
- Coffee. I love it, but only in the morning for that caffeine jolt. It loses its magic if you drink it all day. Just so you know,

cold-brewed organic coffee is less acidic than regular coffee. If you like regular coffee, go for organic/Fair Trade varieties and skip the conventional sweeteners and dairy. (I like my coffee black and strong.) Use natural sugars and dairy-free milk such as coconut, almond, or hemp.

- Dark leafy greens, either in whole form or juiced. They're loaded with vitamins, minerals, and micronutrients.
- Ginger shot with lemon and cayenne pepper. This will wake you up in a hurry!
- Maca. A Peruvian root that has been used for thousands of years to increase energy levels, maca is especially good at boosting your body's natural hormone production and fertility. It's also an adaptogen (which helps the body in adapting to stress) and increases energy, improves mood stabilization, and boosts libido in men and women. (Please note: Women who are pregnant or breast-feeding should avoid taking maca.)
- Matcha tea. This is a highly concentrated green tea that is a terrific metabolism booster.
- Yerba maté tea. This tea is made from the leaves of a South American holly tree, and is often drunk by locals instead of coffee for a morning wakeup; it provides slow and steady energy and has more caffeine than tea but less than coffee.

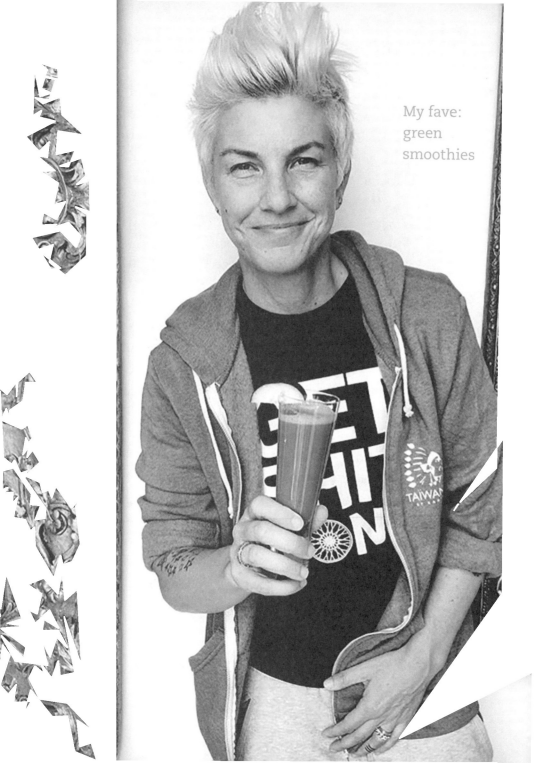

My fave:
green
smoothies

# THE BEST ENERGIZING FOODS TO CONSUME BEFORE A WORKOUT

I have students who love to eat a full meal before coming to class, while others have eaten dinner the night before a morning class, but don't eat right before class. I know a marathon runner who eats an enormous peanut butter and jelly sandwich before every hour-long training session and never has a burp. But that is so *not* me! I am not a fan of eating very much—and certainly never a large meal—before a workout. It's best to keep the stomach as empty as you can stand it and allow your energy to go toward your muscles instead of your digestive system. In yoga and meditation practices, it's also best to eat afterward. (My pro-athlete friend Conor Dwyer religiously has chocolate milk after his Olympic training sessions. Go figure!)

That said, if I wake up really hungry, I'll have a small glass of overnight oats (the recipe is later in this chapter), or grab a banana and a black coffee and drink a lot of water before I start teaching at seven thirty A.M. Although I don't ride when I'm teaching, I still expend a tremendous amount of mental and physical energy, and need to be primed for these workouts. (I burn the same calories when I teach as I would if I were on a bike—dancing and concentrating so hard have their benefits!) I'll choose from any of these:

- Water (preferably filtered), with a teaspoon or so of raw honey or maple syrup and the juice of one lemon.

- Coconut water (preferably fresh—from Juice Press or Harmless Harvest, found at Whole Foods or your local health-food store).
- Small smoothie (fresh coconut-based).
- If I'm very hungry, I have a snack of low-sugar fresh fruit (ideally, seasonal and local): grapefruit, oranges, or clementines, which I especially love as they fit in your pockets, so they're great when you're on the go (winter/spring); berries (summer); apples or pears (fall /winter); and avocado (year-round).

## THE BEST BRAIN FOODS

The following are foods containing compounds that help with proper brain functioning, giving it the steady stream of nutrients it needs. Did you know your brain is 60 percent fat? It literally cannot function without the fat that gives it energy and helps protect against degenerative brain diseases. Healthy fat is really good for you.

### Fruits and Vegetables

These fruits and veggies are especially high in vitamins, phytonutrients, and antioxidants.

- Avocado
- Beets
- Black currants
- Blueberries
- Broccoli
- Celery
- Spinach
- Sweet potatoes
- Tomatoes

## Proteins

Look for foods high in essential fatty acids, which are critical to optimal brain functioning.

- Oily fish, such as herring, mackerel, salmon, sardines, and trout
- Nuts and seeds, such as chia, flax, hemp, pumpkin, sunflower, and walnuts (raw is best)

## Grains

All whole grains have a low glycemic index, which means they release glucose slowly into your bloodstream, avoiding those spikes triggered by junk carbs that make you irritable and starving soon after you eat. Don't got overboard with them, though, as they can be hard to digest and assimilate.

## Healthy Fats

Your brain (and body) will thank you!

- Avocado
- Coconut oil
- Olive oil (preferably raw or cold pressed)

## Other

Keep these on hand.

- Turmeric. This bright orange spice is well known for its anti-inflammatory effects and may boost the regeneration of brain cells. Sprinkle some on your food.
- Water. Dehydration affects cognitive functioning that can impair focus and short-term memory. Drink water all day long, but preferably not with meals, as this will inhibit proper digestion.

## THE BEST CALMING FOODS

Foods containing potent minerals such as magnesium and calcium help calm the nervous system and relax muscles. They also have an overall sedative effect; they contain B vitamins, which support healthy brain cells and nerve function, and tryptophan, an amino acid that can help boost the levels of serotonin, one of your brain's neurotransmitters that affects your moods and is necessary for that chill factor you're striving to get. Always try to eat foods that are local, seasonal, and non-GMO, as they contain higher levels of nutrients and fewer pesticides and herbicides.

- Avocado. It contains grounding monounsaturated fats and stress-relieving B vitamins. As you'll see in the recipe section at the end of this chapter, this is my favorite go-to snack. I love half an avocado with lemon and pepper.
- Coconut water. It's extremely hydrating and mineralizing, and is an incredible source of magnesium and potassium.
- Dark leafy greens, especially chard and spinach. Their chlorophyll (the "blood" of plants) contains high amounts of magnesium.
- Healthy fats. Good fats like coconut oil, olive oil, or a pat of grass-fed butter increase the nourishing and calming effect of whatever else you're eating.
- Pumpkin seeds, raw. You only need ¼ cup to give you 48 percent of your daily magnesium requirement.
- Root vegetables. Energy-wise, anything that grows in the ground, especially burdock root, carrots, jicama, parsnips, radishes (especially daikon), sweet potatoes, turnips, and yams, has calming, "grounding" properties.
- Salmon. This fish contains protein (amino acids), B vitamins, magnesium, brain-protectiing omega-3 fatty acids, and tryptophan.

- Teas. These teas are known for their calming effect: chamomile, holy basil (also reduces stress), lemon balm, mint, and passion flower (also reduces restlessness and anxiety). I happen to live for Teavana Oprah Chai tea. It's magnificent!
- Vanilla bean. This spice has been used medicinally for hundreds of years. Its earthy, sweet scent is soothing and anxiety-reducing. Try adding a dash to your smoothies.

## THE BEST FOODS TO HELP YOU SLEEP OR NAP

I always try to avoid eating before bedtime, as sleeping on a full stomach inhibits digestion and can give you some very weird dreams! Try to have your last meal of the day at least two hours before bedtime.

Choose any of the foods on the Calming list, above, and add these to them as sleep/relaxation aids:

- Honey (raw). Add 1 teaspoon to one of the calming herbal teas I list or to a cup of nut or seed milk warmed on the stove. (You can make your own nut milk using my recipe on page 256, or buy it fresh at health-food stores or at a juice bar like Juice Press.) Doing this and drinking one of the beverages a few hours before bed will help you unwind. Also, the small amount of glucose from honey lowers orexin, a neurotransmitter that is responsible for alertness. I learned this the hard way, as I used to sometimes eat a bit of raw honey between classes, thinking the natural sugar would give me a jolt of energy, and instead it did the opposite. I couldn't understand why until Meredith told me about the orexin. When in doubt, do your research!

- Tryptophan-rich foods. Tryptophan is an amino acid that has sedative effects, and is found in:
  - Cheese. I love cheese, but I also know that it's a calorie-dense food with no fiber, so it's very easy to eat a lot of it without realizing it, unless it's very pungent. Stick to small servings, which can be hard since cheese is actually addictive; it contains casein, the protein found in milk, that when digested releases an opiate that has an effect on dopamine receptors in the brain responsible for cravings! If you're trying to wean yourself off a cheese addiction, raw cheeses are best, especially those made from goat's or sheep's milk.
  - Eggs, especially the yolks.
  - Nuts and seeds (raw). They are full of protein, good fats, vitamins and minerals, and other trace nutrients. (Just be careful with quantity, as they are calorie-dense.)
  - Tahini (raw). Sesame seeds naturally contain high levels of tryptophan, and are more powerful when raw. Have 1 tablespoon on its own or add a little raw honey.
  - Turkey. Yes, you likely already know this is why you get sleepy on Thanksgiving!
  - Whole grains, especially buckwheat, millet, quinoa, and wild rice. Sprouted versions are ideal. They're best when

Yes, I know this is a chapter about food, but I have to mention how important it is to keep your armor shiny. As in, your skin.

Your skin is your coat, and you need to take care of it. That means eating well, because your skin needs good fats to keep it looking plump and dewy, and the antioxidants in fruit and veggies to help protect it from environmental assault; getting enough sleep, so you look refreshed; and to do what my mom taught me—which is to never, ever leave the house without wearing sunscreen.

I'm a California girl, and my skin looks as good as it does because I've always kept it protected from the sun's harmful radiation. Even when I was an addict, I took extremely good care of my skin and body. I put on sunscreen with an SPF of 30 or 50. I apply it when I'm brushing my teeth in the morning so I don't forget—and I also know that it takes up to twenty minutes to activate.

If I'm out in the sun, I use a *shitload* of broad-spectrum sunscreen and I reapply it all the time. I wear a hat and sunglasses sometimes, too, but always with the 50 on. No way am I gonna get burned! I've found that for me at least, the deepest, darkest, sun-kissed skin comes from wearing sunscreen at SPF 45 or more. Your tan will also stay longer.

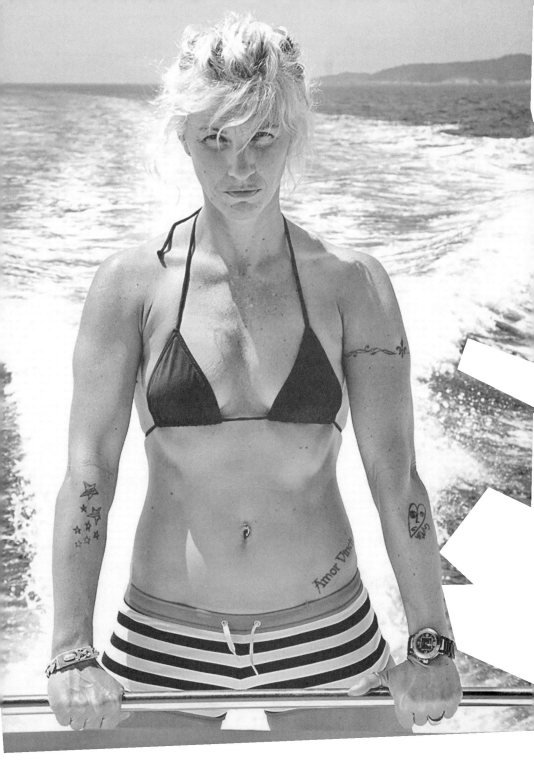

combined with low-starch vegetables such as dark leafy greens because this will assist proper digestion and assimilation.

## THE BEST FOODS TO AWAKEN OR HIGHLIGHT YOUR SENSUALITY

When you're looking to juice up your libido, these foods have aphrodisiac properties thanks to their high levels of iron, which helps oxygenate the blood; vitamins A, C, E, and beta-carotene, which are antioxidants; and magnesium, which helps in the production of sex hormones and promotes heart health. Choose any from this list:

- Avocado. The Aztecs were the first documented culture to eat avocados, and they considered this fruit to be an aphrodisiac based on its appearance. Avocados are rich in vitamin E (often referred to as the "sex vitamin"), which helps maintain youthful vigor.
- Basil. This fragrant herb has historically been used by women as a scent of seduction, and that's why it's used in many perfume formulations (and pesto!).
- Cacao. Cacao contains properties that stimulate parts of the brain responsible for creating pleasurable sensations, and boosts serotonin and endorphin levels as well. The naturally occurring elements in chocolate can mimic the feeling

of being in love. It is also very high in magnesium.

- Cayenne. This spicy pepper encourages blood flow to the body's most sensitive areas.
- Ginger. Same as cayenne. It's also very soothing.
- Rosemary. Did you know that Aphrodite, the goddess of love, was born and rose from the sea wearing rosemary around her neck? Sexy goddess! This herb boosts blood supply, increases skin's sensitivity, and has an intoxicating aroma. It contains loads of vitamins and nutrients that aid in boosting libido and sexual performance, especially for men.

## THE MOST IMPORTANT FOOD TO AVOID

No, it's not fat. It's *sugar*. Why did people gain so much weight when they started eating fat-free foods? Because the fat was replaced with sugar! Worse, in September 2016 it was revealed in the journal *JAMA Internal Medicine* that the Sugar Association paid researchers at Harvard in the 1960s to downplay the effects of sugar on heart disease, and shift the blame to fat instead. If lobbyists can sway the medical profession, how can consumers know who to trust?

Whenever you eat any kind of carbohydrate—a large category that includes all dairy, fruit, legumes (beans, lentils, and soy), nuts and seeds, starches (grains, potatoes), sugars, and, yes, even healthy, low-calorie vegetables—your pancreas re-

Do you know why you should always trust your gut feelings? Not only due to the power of intuition, but because so much communication goes on between our digestive systems and our brains. You have ten times more bacteria in your gut than you do human cells, by the way! Researchers are only beginning to understand how this process works, but the bottom line for us right now is that you need to ensure you have the healthiest gut possible, with your microbiome, or thriving colonies of the more than five hundred species of beneficial bacteria that are essential for proper digestion and nutrient absorption.

You could be eating the best diet possible, but if your gut isn't working well, you're not going to reap the benefits. If you're out of whack (which you know can easily happen if you take antibiotics for an infection—not only do they kill the toxic bacteria making you sick, but the good gut bacteria, too, leaving you with diarrhea or other problems), you need to replenish the flora as quickly as possible. When your beneficial bacteria, or microflora, levels are thriving, you'll have more energy, more brain power, and fewer cravings for junk food or snacking.

One of the easiest ways to ensure good gut health is with probiotics. These are different strains of some of the most common, beneficial bacteria your gut needs. We can get probiotics from food as well as in supplement form, and I recommend you do both.

## FOOD WITH PROBIOTICS

- Yogurt. Choose plain yogurt, as the sweetened varieties are overloaded with sugars. Greek yogurt has a higher protein content and is much more satisfying and filling. Coconut yogurt is an excellent alternative if you're trying to avoid dairy. (Raw yogurt has the highest probiotic levels, but selling raw dairy is illegal in most states.)

• Fermented foods are some of the best things you can eat. During fermentation, the immersion of food into a salty brine kills off bad bacteria while allowing good bacteria like *Lactobacillus* and *Bifidobacterium* to thrive, and it also helps to break down lactose sugars and starches—which is why a fermented dairy item like kefir is easier to digest and better for you than milk. The best fermented foods are dark chocolate (yay!), fresh kefir (drinkable yogurt, which has a much higher probiotic count than regular yogurt; be careful, though, with store-bought varieties that can contain a lot of sugar and fillers), kimchi (spicy Korean fermented cabbage), miso (fermented Japanese grains), pickles (fermented cucumbers or other veggies), sauerkraut (fermented cabbage), tempeh (fermented soy protein), and wheatgrass (which has naturally occurring probiotics and should only be consumed when fresh, not frozen, and when juiced). Note: Fermented foods ideally should be consumed within the first seven days of fermentation. After that, the food turns into lactic acid. So freshly made kimchi, sauerkraut, pickles, and kefir are ideal.

## PROBIOTIC SUPPLEMENTS

This is now a popular category on vitamin shelves, but it's easy to waste your money with little benefits if you choose one that can't survive the acids in your stomach—which most can't. The brand Meredith and I recommend is Proviotic by Juice Press. It has the added benefit of being vegan. Meredith also likes Earth Biotics as well as Friendly Force by Health Force Nutritionals, in capsule or powder form (the powder can be blended in homemade smoothies), and Threelac or PB8 for travel. Note: Probiotics should always be taken on an empty stomach (first thing in the morning is ideal). Also, it's important to alternate with different strains to improve their efficacy.

leases insulin, the hormone responsible for regulating your blood sugar and keeping it at steady levels.

Complex carbohydrates, such as fiber-rich veggies and beans, as well as proteins, do not trigger an insulin spike. Sugars and starches, which are simple carbohydrates, do. But starches are not the enemy, especially complex starches such as whole grains and starchier veggies (yams, sweet potato, beets). Even a baked white potato (organic only, because conventional potatoes are loaded with pesticides and herbicides) is unfairly linked with processed white foods such as white pasta and white bread. (Note: A *baked* potato is *not* a plate of french fries!) In fact, if you don't have blood sugar issues, white potatoes contain high levels of mineral salts and when cooked properly are healthier and a much cleaner food to eat than even whole grains! It is best to consume all starchier veggies with water-containing greens, such as green leafy salads or cooked greens, for easier digestion, absorption, assimilation, and elimination.

Sugar, on the other hand, causes an immediate insulin surge. The more sugar you ingest, the more insulin is released, which then causes your blood sugar to go down, which in turn sends a signal to your brain that you need more fuel. The result? You feel a desperate need to eat. This explains why having a large bowl of sweetened cereal and a piece of toast for breakfast will leave you hungry an hour or two later.

Worse, if you eat more calories of simple carbs than your body can metabolize, the sugars are converted to a substance stored in your cells for use at some point in the future. That substance is *fat*.

The problem with sugar runs deeper than just insulin and blood sugar spikes. Too much sugar stresses the liver and pancreas, which are the two organs responsible for detoxifying your body. It also creates inflammation, which scientists now believe is an integral component of triggering many autoimmune disorders. It also raises cholesterol levels, offsets the healthy bacteria in your gut, and ages your skin. Combined with unhealthy fats and starches, sugar becomes even more deadly, especially for those who are at an unhealthy weight due to a diet overloaded with packaged and junk foods.

On its own, not only is sugar devoid of nutrients, protein, enzymes, and healthy fats, but it's an incredibly addictive substance that raises the levels of serotonin and dopamine, the brain's feel-good chemicals, leaving you always wanting more and never feeling satisfied no matter how much you consume. Some studies have even shown that sugar is eight times more addictive than cocaine.

This is one of the reasons America is suffering from an unprecedented obesity crisis, in people of all ages, leading to an enormous upswing not just in preventable conditions such as hypertension, metabolic syndrome, and fatty liver syndrome, but in life-threatening diseases like type 2 diabetes, heart disease, and some cancers.

Bottom line: Sugar is toxic. Overconsumption of sugar can literally kill you. According to the American Heart Association, women should have no more than 100 calories and men no more than 150 calories every day from added sugar in their diet. That's less than one can of soda!

Of all the sugars, two are particularly bad. Refined sugar, or sucrose, is made from beets or sugar cane, and includes white and brown sugars. It is a simple sugar made from glucose molecules. High-fructose corn syrup comes from corn, and is particularly dangerous as it contains fructose as well as glucose; fructose is metabolized directly by your liver, making it particularly unhealthy.

One more thing—replacing sugar-laden foods with artificially sweetened foods doesn't work. When your body realizes something sweet has been ingested, it responds with an insulin release, even if it's a fake sugar. This is why people who drink a lot of diet soda often have a very hard time losing weight.

Believe me, I know how hard it is to kick the sugar habit. It's ingrained in us, right? We're taught from that very first slice of our very first birthday cake at our very first birthday party that getting something sweet is a reward. Sugar was the dessert we could have only as a reward for eating our broccoli. Sugar was our reward at any celebration.

So in order to cut down on sugar, you need to change your reward system, and stop associating dessert or candy with a present you give your sweet tooth. If you're a sugar addict, don't try to go cold turkey. Slowly cut back. Have a lot more fruit on hand at first. I know it's hard to believe, but once you stop eating so much sugar, you will lose your taste for it, and what you once ate mindlessly will suddenly strike you as completely unpalatable.

You can also try to eat like the French. They rarely have a sweet dessert—instead, they'll have salad and then a few very small pieces of cheese with, perhaps, a pear or an apple after their main course. They know that eating something extremely pungent and flavorful cleanses their palate and kills the cravings for sweets. In addition, the typical French breakfast of a tartine—a piece of fresh baguette with butter and jam—along with a yogurt and a café au lait is like having dessert for breakfast.

---

SG TRUTH  **No wonder I used sugar so much when I got sober—it became my new crack. It also explains why I was twenty pounds heavier!**

---

## WHAT TO DO WHEN CRAVINGS HIT

It happens to all of us. Maybe you go for sweets like candy, or maybe you go for savory like potato chips or mashed potatoes—but whatever your craving food, it's awfully hard to resist, especially if you've had a rotten day and need something that you

Beware of hidden sugars—it's amazing how many packaged food items are laden with totally unnecessary sugars to make them taste better. Do you really need sugar in your peanut butter? Or pasta sauce? Or ketchup? Or frozen microwave meal? Of course not.

Be a smart consumer and scour food labels before you buy anything. A package might say "organic raw cane sugar," but guess what? It's still sugar. Take a good look at this list—it's shocking how many different types of sugars there are:

| | | |
|---|---|---|
| Agave | Fructose | Malt sugar |
| Barley malt | Fruit sugars | Mannitol |
| Beet sugar | Glucose | Maple sugar |
| Brown rice syrup | Glucose polymers | (Blackstrap) molasses |
| Brown sugar | High-fructose corn syrup | Monk fruit |
| Cane sugar | Honey | Sorbitol |
| Coconut nectar | Invert sugar | Stevia |
| Coconut palm sugar | Lactose | Sucanat |
| Corn syrup | Maltitol | Turbinado sugar |
| Date sugar | Maltodextrin | Yacon syrup |
| Dextrose | Maltose | Xylitol |

know always makes you feel better in the moment (even if it makes you feel awful *after* you've eaten it!).

That's when you're most at risk for a Snack Attack.

One of my weaknesses is Hebrew National hot dogs with sauerkraut. I smell one and it is very hard to resist. Before

## WHAT SUGARS ARE HEALTHIER SUBSTITUTES?

Obviously, a life devoid of all sweet-tasting food isn't feasible or realistic. If you're going to have something sweet, enjoy every last morsel. Feeling guilty over eating something is a waste of time and energy. Just enjoy it! A small square of raw dark chocolate, for example, is loaded with antioxidants and phytonutrients, and it's satisfying to both the body and soul.

The following sugars are better for you than white table sugar or, especially, high-fructose corn syrup. Try to buy organic sweeteners whenever possible, too:

Coconut nectar

Coconut palm sugar

Date sugar

Dates (whole, raw, unsulfured)

Figs (whole, raw, unsulfured)

Maple syrup (grade B, which is less processed)

Molasses (blackstrap only)

Monk fruit

Raw honey (be careful when selecting, as some of the cheaper honeys are really just sugar!)

Stevia (the powdered form is less processed, or liquid)

Yacon syrup (made from a root found in South America)

Xylitol

Also try using spices like cinnamon; on their own, they aren't sweet, but your taste buds associate them with sweet things so they make you think they are. Even better, cinnamon also lowers your blood sugar.

scarfing it down, I have to ask myself: Am I really hungry for this snack? Or am I thirsty/bored/frustrated/stuck? Is my brain telling me to do something interesting so I can avoid dealing with what's *really* going on, or am I legit hungry?

---

**SG TRUTH** I usually have at least six over the summer months, so I figure six hot dogs out of 365 days is pretty good!

---

These tips will help you manage your cravings.

## Before Reaching for Food

- Often, when you think you're hungry, you're really just thirsty. Sip water or tea. My favorite Urge Surfer is hot water with lemon. I drink it all day sometimes, even when it's really hot outside. It detoxes your liver and makes me feel clean and fresh. You can get an electric kettle that heats water up very quickly, so you don't have to stand around in the kitchen and wonder what to eat while waiting for the water to boil.

- If you're the kind of person who likes to eat little pieces of things such as M&M's or potato chips, training your mouth means training your fingers, too. These substitutions will help: chewing gum, sugarless hard candy, cough drops, mouthwash, or cut-up tiny pieces of veggies like celery or peppers. Frozen grapes are good, too, because you have to suck on them for a while to melt them so they're soft enough to chew.

- Breathe! Taking three or four long, deep breaths calms the nervous system and allows you to take a pause before launching into the snacks.

- If you have the time and are at home, soak. An Epsom salt bath is loaded with magnesium and helps curb cravings. (You can also try my Spiritual Bath products, as they are amazing!) A shower can work, too.
- Check in with yourself. Ask, "What am I really craving right now? Is it really food or something else? Am I wanting to eat because I'm bored or frustrated?"
- Give yourself a jolt. Do twenty jumping jacks. March around the room. Take the dog for a walk. Return the phone call you've been putting off.

## When You Really *Are* Hungry

Be prepared! Have the following items available when cravings hit.

- Fresh green juice. Try carrot-apple if you don't like greens. This will alkalinize your body, which in turn will cut cravings. Trust me—you will be amazed at the results!
- 1 tablespoon truly raw honey. Local is best. Eat the honey very slowly. I also like manuka honey, which is found only in New Zealand and is more medicinal in nature as it has antiviral and antibacterial properties. (It is an acquired taste and is also very expensive.)
- Healthy fats. These are very filling and satisfying. My go-to food when I am really hungry and in need of a snack is half an avocado with a little fresh lemon juice and pepper. I only

add a bit of sea salt if I have just worked out, and eat it out of the skin with a spoon. Or try 1 tablespoon raw organic coconut oil or coconut butter.

- Make smart swaps. If you're craving a burger, have one—with lettuce leaves instead of a bun. Have a veggie burger (some brands really do taste just like chicken, too, but be wary of the lesser brands that contain fillers, soy, and sugars).
- Berries. As I said already, we always keep small bowls of berries on a shelf in the fridge, next to bottles of water, so they're all right there when I open the door and I can grab whatever I want. They're also good frozen.
- If you want a bit of crunch, go for celery or carrot sticks or cucumber slices. They're much better than crackers to dip into your avocado.
- Nuts in the shell. This is a great trick when you get the craving for crunch, as it not only makes the craving go away, but keeps your hands busy so you can't eat anything else—I did this when I was trying to quit smoking (and it worked). Buy yourself a really nice handheld nutcracker. Keep your hard-shelled nuts in a lovely bowl. Then get cracking.
- A baked sweet potato. Add sea salt and a bit of lemon juice or spicy mustard.
- A small bowl of a fermented vegetable. Try sauerkraut, kimchi, or pickles. They are very flavorful and have almost no calories.
- A small square of raw chocolate. My favorite brand is called Sinless (it figures!).

- Chocolate tea. A brand called Numi makes an incredible Chocolate Pu-erh tea that makes you feel like you're eating food when you're drinking it.

If you do have a Snack Attack, don't beat yourself up. As I've said already, enjoy what you've eaten. Work out harder the next day. Don't tell yourself that you're bad or hopeless. Change your reward system—one that tells you that your reward is giving your body the healthy eating it needs and deserves, especially if you've been exercising a lot or performing anything at a high level. That's the best reward there is.

Then set your intentions and make different choices tomorrow. You can start over every time you blink your eyes. You don't need to wait until the first of the month, a Monday, or a specific birthday. You can change your eating patterns *now*! Just make sure that once you decide to make the change, you give yourself an actual time frame to "eat clean." Most of the time you do . . . sometimes you don't . . . focus on the *most of the time*, and you'll be fine.

## HOW I EAT NOW

As with many people, life slowly became more complex and a whole lot busier as years went by. Between work, family, and social life, I became more and more exhausted—not something I was used to, as my energy level had always been high.

I had become more reliant on comfort food, making bad choices when I was starving in the middle of the day from not having breakfast, teaching several classes, and running to meetings.

And then at night, when I was too tired to cook, there was the pitfall known to all New Yorkers: the takeout menu. With free delivery and endless specials. Then I would get bummed about my crummy eating habits, my body not looking its best despite all my daily physical exertion, my mind not as focused despite all my teaching, the bags under my eyes deepening because I wasn't getting enough deep sleep, and my stomach rebelling from all the recommended supplements I was scarfing. My anemia, which I've been prone to all my life, got so extreme, my doctor had to put me on iron infusions.

Did I listen to my body? Did I consult a nutritionist? No, I did not. I did what nearly everyone else I knew did—I self-diagnosed my food issues. Was it middle age? Not enough sleep? Stress? Fried food? Contrary to what I knew was sound medical advice, I signed up for some of those all-too-popular juice cleanses. They worked at first, so I tried juicing until dinner and then eating a healthy meal. Both of these options left me irritable and insatiably hungry. You can guess what happened next. I went right back to my same bad eating habits and issues.

Something had to give, and that something became my diet.

Let me tell you how this all changed, almost overnight—and I wouldn't believe it if I hadn't lived through it. My girlfriend had a lot of the same symptoms that I did, and was searching for explanations and help as well. One night, she stumbled upon a community on Instagram that changed everything. It was called "The Healthy Foodies," a healthy eating site devoted to sharing blogs, websites, recommendations, clean living, and recipes, compiled by an incredible woman named Sonia. And there I was, always trying to minimize my social media.

---

**SG TRUTH** I do love cleansing in a pinch to lose three to six pounds, especially if I have a photo shoot, an event, or feel the need to kick-start something.

---

She started following some of the Instagram accounts and their blogs, fascinated by all the stories of life-changing healthy diets she was reading about. They were written by real women, discussing vegan, vegetarian, Paleo and non-Paleo, and just healthy lifestyles and eating habits. This was the missing link. I've always said what you eat is the gas that fuels your motor. But I didn't realize just how critical this link is.

So we completely changed our eating habits. We don't label our eating into any specific category, but pull from many. We no longer order in, choosing to cook most of our meals instead. I think one of the most important notes from our new way of eating is, don't let cooking intimidate you. The unknown can seem overwhelming, but like anything else . . . if I can rise to the challenge, so can you!

Take a week or two, or three, and get comfortable with your kitchen, tools, appliances, and new ingredients. Make shopping lists, and use them. Plan ahead, even if it's only by one day. I was astonished when I saw how little time it actually took my girlfriend to make what became some of my favorite recipes, and leftovers can taste even better than a dish did the first time. Have some friends over when you're cooking new recipes for the first time, and make it an impromptu party.

**SG TRUTH** I don't do any of the cooking. I sit in a chair by the kitchen door with the dogs and watch my love pivot from side to side, cooking up a storm. We enjoy this time so much together; it's become a bonding experience, and one of the favorite moments of my day.

Get creative and experiment. Make it your own—and have fun. You're not only going to watch your food bills go way down, but you're going to be making a sound investment in your body's health and strength.

Remember—food is power. You need it to think, perform, love, breathe, sleep, and exist. You truly are what you eat!

## What I Typically Eat During the Day

I teach twenty classes a week and am in perpetual motion. I need to keep eating and drinking (and napping!) in order to be the best possible teacher. This is what fuels me on a typical day.

### Breakfast

I am not a breakfast person and usually don't eat it unless we're on vacation (in which case I'll go for a fruit bowl). When I'm teaching, I usually have a large bottle of water and a banana.

My students often ask me how I can have so much energy early in the morning, especially when I'm not into breakfast, and I tell them it's because I had a good dinner the night before and a really good night's sleep. If you're like me and truly not hungry in the morning, don't force yourself to eat breakfast just because many experts say it's the most important meal of the day. For a lot of people, it is. If so, go for it. If you have blood sugar issues, it is especially important to eat when you get up, particularly a meal with a lot of fiber, complex carbs, protein, and some fat.

Try a bowl of steel-cut oats or quinoa with a small slice of cheese on top for some extra protein, or Greek yogurt on the side. Or a slice of whole-grain toast with peanut butter or real butter and slices of banana. Or loaded avocado toast. What you should never eat is a bagel with a schmear, or a bowl of sweetened cereal, or *anything* sweet and/or junk food. That will send your blood sugar shooting out into the stratosphere, and you'll crash a short time later as your brain screams for more fuel.

### Lunch

I teach until eleven thirty A.M., and for lunch will usually have a protein shake with kale and apple.

### Dinner

I'll have a home-cooked meal with a balance of protein and carbs. I love white fish baked in parchment paper on a bed of jasmine rice with tomato. Mmm!

### Snacks

I try to avoid snacks, sometimes unsuccessfully, but I try. Instead of eating, I'll have lots of fresh Vitamixed juices and water all day. I tend to have walnuts handy, but don't eat too many as they are hard for me to digest.

## A Sample Week of Our Healthy Eating

*Recipe included

### Monday

BREAKFAST
Overnight Oats* (this can also be an early lunch if you're not a big breakfast eater)

LUNCH OR SNACK
Stacey Smoothie* (make extra and put in freezer in ice pop molds)

SNACK *(if you didn't eat lunch)*
Brown rice cakes with all-natural almond or peanut butter and raspberry or blueberry chia jam

DINNER
Quinoa with roasted vegetables, topped with crispy kale (optional:
top with poached or over-easy runny egg)

## Tuesday

LUNCH
Butternut squash soup with crispy leeks and toasted pumpkin or
sunflower seeds

SNACK
Stacey Smoothie*

DINNER
Gray sole in parchment paper with cherry tomatoes, over small bed
of jasmine rice

## Wednesday

LUNCH
Overnight oats with peanut butter and jelly

SNACK
Stacey Smoothie*

DINNER
Chicken Milanese on bed of arugula with cherry tomatoes

## Thursday

LUNCH
Out with friends

SNACK
Matcha tea granola with rolled oats, buckwheat groats, and goji
berries

DINNER
Stuffed baked sweet potato on bed of quinoa

## Friday

**LUNCH**
Brown rice with roasted vegetables, grilled firm tofu with sesame
seeds and cashew cream sauce

**DINNER**
Pasta Three Ways*

## Saturday

**BREAKFAST**
Avocado Toast Galore*

**SNACK**
Crunchy peanut butter bars

**DINNER**
Would be our night out at a restaurant. If not, it's our special steak
night, made in a cast-iron skillet, with baked fries.

## Sunday

**BREAKFAST**
Steel-Cut Oats*

**SNACK**
Lots of watermelon triangles and clementines

**DINNER**
Massaman chicken or veggie curry over bed of jasmine rice

## TOOLS

Cast-iron or nonstick skillet

Cookie sheets

Cutting boards

Food processor

Grater/slicer

Measuring cups and spoons

Nonreactive pots and pans,
including a large soup pot

Knives—This is one tool where
you can't skimp. Get a really
good set.

Strainer and fine strainer

Vitamix—This blender is the bomb,
but it is very expensive. You do
need a blender, so pick one that's
sturdy and powerful and fits your
budget.

Tongs

Wooden or rubber spoons

## FOOD ITEMS

Berries—Keep them in little
bowls in the fridge so you
snack on them instead
of candy.

Coconut oil

Extra-virgin olive oil

Herbs and spices—
Buy small quantities
so they stay fresh.

Greek yogurt

Maple syrup or honey

Mustard

Nuts—Use cashews or almonds to
make your own nut milk.

Palm sugar

Rolled oats and steel-cut oats

Sea salt

Vinegar

KITCHEN MUST-HAVES

## MY FAVORITE RECIPES

These are the go-to recipes for me and my girlfriend. They're not only super nutritious, but super filling and super easy, too.

## BREAKFAST
# Avocado Toast Galore

Pesto sauce (optional)
1 slice of toasted sourdough bread, or 1 brown rice cake
A few arugula leaves
$\frac{1}{2}$ lemon
Extra-virgin olive oil or coconut oil
$\frac{1}{2}$ avocado, sliced
1 egg, cooked to your preference
Seasonings of your choice

1. If desired, spread a thin layer of pesto on the bread.
2. Layer on arugula.
3. Squeeze most of the lemon juice over it. Drizzle on a bit of olive or coconut oil
4. Top with the avocado slices.
5. Place the egg carefully on top.
6. Season with some of your favorites: sunflower seeds, red pepper flakes, paprika, salt and black pepper, and the rest of the lemon juice.

# Overnight Oats

**This needs to be started the night before you want to eat it.**

²/₃ cup rolled oats (*not* instant)
1 teaspoon chia seeds
¹/₄ cup frozen raspberries (see Note)
¹/₄ cup frozen strawberries
1 teaspoon raw almond or peanut butter
1 to 3 teaspoons pure maple syrup
¹/₂ to 1 cup nut milk or pressed apple juice
Toppings of your choice

1.  Choose your favorite glass tumbler or mason jar. Line the bottom with ¹/₃ cup of the rolled oats. Top with the chia seeds.

2.  Add the raspberries and strawberries.

3.  Add the almond or peanut butter.

4.  Pour on the maple syrup (more if you like it very sweet; I only use a little).

5.  Top with the remaining ¹/₃ cup oats.

6.  Pour the nut milk or pressed apple juice over all the ingredients to fill the jar.

7.  Cover with plastic wrap or a lid and refrigerate overnight.

8.  In the morning, add your favorite toppings (granola, more nut butter, chia jam, pomegranate seeds, flax seeds, cashew cream, and smoothies are some of my favorites).

Note: You can use any fruit you like. Try passion fruit mango, or blackberries instead of the raspberries and strawberries.

# Cashew Cream/Cashew Milk

**Experiment with how much water you add to the nuts, as less water makes a thicker cream, and more water makes a thinner milk. You really don't need to measure the nuts.**

Raw cashews
Cold water

1. In a large bowl or pitcher, soak raw cashew nuts overnight in enough cold water to completely submerge them.

2. In the morning, drain the nuts and put them in a blender with fresh filtered water and blend to the desired thickness. Add more or less water as desired.

Note: For sweetness and taste you can add 1 to 3 pitted fresh dates to the blender along with a dash of vanilla.

## SNACKS

For all smoothies, make large batches and freeze the extra in ice pop molds.

# Stacey Smoothie #1

1 cup frozen or fresh ripe pineapple
1 frozen banana (see Note)
1 small piece fresh ginger, peeled and sliced
Juice of 1 lemon
1 cup almond milk, fresh orange juice, or coconut water
1 teaspoon ground turmeric
Pinch of black pepper

Combine all the ingredients in a high-speed blender and blend until smooth. Add a few ice cubes if the fruit is not frozen.

Note: To freeze bananas, wait for the bananas to fully ripen, break them into four sections, and wrap in parchment paper, then store in the freezer until ready to use in smoothies. Or you can mash them up and freeze them that way, too.

## Stacey Smoothie #2

1 cup almond milk

$1/2$ cup frozen strawberries

1 frozen banana (see Note, above)

1 tablespoon chia seeds

1 to 2 tablespoons raw cacao powder

1 teaspoon to 1 tablespoon pure maple syrup

Combine all the ingredients in a high-speed blender and blend until smooth.

## Stacey Smoothie #3

2 big handfuls kale

1 big handful spinach

$1/2$ avocado, pitted and peeled

1 Granny Smith apple, peeled and cored

$1/3$ cucumber, skin on

1 tablespoon ground flaxseed

1 to $1^1/2$ cups cold water or coconut water, depending on desired thickness

Combine all the ingredients in a high-speed blender and blend until smooth.

## BREAKFAST
# Steel-Cut Oats

**This is great for a family-style breakfast or a brunch.**

1 cup steel-cut oats
Toppings: fresh raspberries, blueberries, blackberries, palm
sugar, pure maple syrup, pomegranate seeds, flaxseeds, sliced
almonds, caramelized bananas, sautéed figs or nectarines, loose
granola, cashew cream, ground cinnamon, and/or chia jam

1. Bring 4 cups water to a boil in a saucepan. Add the oatmeal
   and return to a boil.

2. Cook until the mixture becomes smoother and thicker, then
   lower the heat and simmer, stirring occasionally, for 30
   minutes.

3. Set up a smorgasbord of topping options.

4. Place a few ladles of oats in each bowl, then add whatever you
   like from the toppings bar.

## DINNER
# Pasta Three Ways
SERVES 2

## Pasta #1—Roasted Tomato Sauce and Meatballs

**This sauce tastes great the next day, and is easy to double or
triple—so make enough for leftovers. Add extra tomatoes to the
recipe if you like it very saucy!**

10 to 20 cherry tomatoes on the vine, halved

1 tablespoon plus 1 teaspoon extra-virgin olive oil

3 garlic cloves, sliced

Sea salt and black pepper

1 or 2 (14-ounce) cans unsalted diced tomatoes (or use all fresh tomatoes)

1 pound ground turkey, pork, beef, or ground vegetables

1 egg, beaten

1/4 cup unseasoned bread crumbs

Garlic powder

Onion powder

8 ounces dried or fresh pasta (egg, spinach, tomato, gluten-free— whatever works for your diet)

1. Preheat the oven to 375°F.

2. In a bowl, toss the cherry tomatoes with 1 tablespoon of the olive oil, the garlic, and salt and pepper to taste.

3. Spread them on a baking sheet and roast for about 12 minutes, or until the tomatoes have shriveled a bit.

4. Transfer the cherry tomato mixture to a medium saucepan. Add the canned tomatoes, stir well, and heat over low heat.

5. In a bowl, mix the ground meat or veggies with the egg and bread crumbs, and season with salt, pepper, garlic powder, and onion powder. Form into medium-sized balls (about the size of a golf ball).

6. In a saucepan, heat the remaining 1 teaspoon oil over medium heat. Add the meatballs and brown them, turning often to make sure all sides brown evenly.

7. Add the meatballs to the tomato sauce. Bring the sauce to a boil, then reduce the heat to maintain a simmer and cook for at least 1 hour. Stir occasionally, making sure the sauce doesn't stick to the bottom of the pot. *(cont.)*

8. Meanwhile, cook the pasta according to directions on the package until al dente. Drain.

9. Place the pasta in a serving bowl and add the meatballs with as much extra sauce as you prefer.

## Pasta #2—Pesto Sauce

**Use leftover pesto sauce for your weekend Avocado Toasts (page 254).**

2 cups fresh spinach

2 cups fresh basil

¼ cup pine nuts

¼ cup walnuts

3 tablespoons extra-virgin olive oil

2 or 3 garlic cloves

1 to 2 tablespoons grated Parmesan cheese or nutritional yeast,
plus more for serving

Salt and black pepper

Juice of 1 lemon

8 ounces dried fusilli or capellini

1. In a blender, combine the spinach, basil, pine nuts, walnuts, olive oil, garlic, and cheese or nutritional yeast. Blend until well mixed. Stir in salt, pepper, and lemon juice to taste. For thinner pesto, add a bit of water.

2. Cook the pasta according to the package directions until al dente. Drain.

3. Pour the pesto over the hot pasta and stir until well mixed. Top with additional cheese or nutritional yeast, if desired.

## Pasta #3—Spicy Garlic and Oil with Shrimp

**If you want to add veggies, add trimmed Brussels sprouts in step 2.**

¼ cup plus 1 tablespoon extra-virgin olive oil

1 teaspoon sea salt

Pinch of black pepper

5 garlic cloves, thinly sliced

¼ to 1 teaspoon red pepper flakes

4 to 8 raw shrimp, peeled and deveined

8 ounces dried spaghetti or fettuccini

1. In a saucepan, heat ¼ cup of the olive oil with the salt and black pepper over medium-low heat until simmering.

2. Add the garlic and cook for 2 to 3 minutes, until fragrant and golden brown but not burned. Add the red pepper flakes, using more or less to taste, and sauté for 2 minutes more.

3. In a separate pan, heat the remaining 1 tablespoon oil. Add the shrimp and sauté until pink, then transfer the shrimp to the spicy oil and cook for another minute or so to blend the flavors.

4. Meanwhile, cook pasta according to the package directions until al dente. Drain. Pour the sauce on top and enjoy.

"Every body should be a strong body."

# EIGHT
## TRAIN

Everybody says exercise is something they *have* to do. The magic comes when you make it something you *love* to do—and especially when you make working out a tool to change your life.

I'm going to give you the motivation to push yourself into a zone where moving your muscles becomes as vital as brushing your teeth! Think of it as "brush your muscles/brush your teeth!"

You'll crave some kind of motion every day. . . . It's incredibly powerful, because it becomes a part of who you are!

So how do we train your body to get into that zone?

Well, it doesn't just happen with weights or machines or a new pair of running shoes. You get there with your *state of mind*. I know that sounds counterintuitive, but your sense of physicality comes from the way you *think,* not just how you move your muscles (and joints and bones and everything else).

Everybody needs physical power in their lives. You need to be physically connected to your body—it's called physical presence. You gotta move it—or you're gonna lose it.

Knowing how and why exercise so profoundly affects your body and your brain can help you get into that mind-set.

According to Dr. Suzanne Steinbaum, director of Women's Heart Health at the Heart and Vascular Institute at Lenox Hill Hospital in New York and author of *Dr. Suzanne Steinbaum's Heart Book,* "Exercise is by far the best medicine you can take for your health. *Nothing* else can do for your body what exercise does."

You know what else? Dr. Nick Cavill, a public health specialist and research associate at the University of Oxford in the UK, said, "If exercise were a pill, it would be one of the most cost-effective drugs ever invented."

Want proof? Take Isabel, who is one of my favorite students. We just celebrated her seventy-sixth birthday—with a ninety-minute ride! She knows better than anybody that adding movement into your regular routine can change your own world in a day.

Our celebration came at the end of a rough year for Isabel. And I can tell you that if anyone had every legitimate excuse possible to miss my class, she did. It all started with a diagnosis of breast cancer. She needed to have multiple surgeries and that was followed by chemotherapy. That's enough to sock anybody and drain them of the energy we all need to move our bodies.

But Isabel was determined that instead of letting go of exercise during this time, she was going to make it as much a part of her cure as her medical treatments.

She is living proof of what Dr. Cavill said—that if exercise were a prescription, every doctor would give it to his or her patients. (Informed doctors, like Dr. Steinbaum, regularly prescribe exercise for many of their patients—and I'm here to fill those prescriptions! I certainly wish more of them would do so.) I know from firsthand experience that exercise is the best medicine you can give yourself for whatever is ailing you, as well as to keep you strong, fit, and on an even keel.

I'm happy to report that Isabel is doing well and still comes to class to kick ass four times a week, without fail!

Francesca is another of my longtime friends and students. She's eighty-four years old and going strong, and began working out with me when she was in her mid-sixties. Franny and I became so close that when her slumlord kicked her out of her apartment, she came and lived with me for three months. This woman is inspiration, spunk, and determination all rolled into one person. She's also living proof that exercise kept her alive during those awful months of not knowing where or how she would keep on living. It is still amazing to me the Franny can ride that bike. She is ninety-seven pounds of lean muscle!

While I'm sure you know how exercise helps you maintain healthy weight loss, and makes you look and feel better, it's just as important to believe that it makes you *feel* better, too. Let's dig into some detail about why that happens.

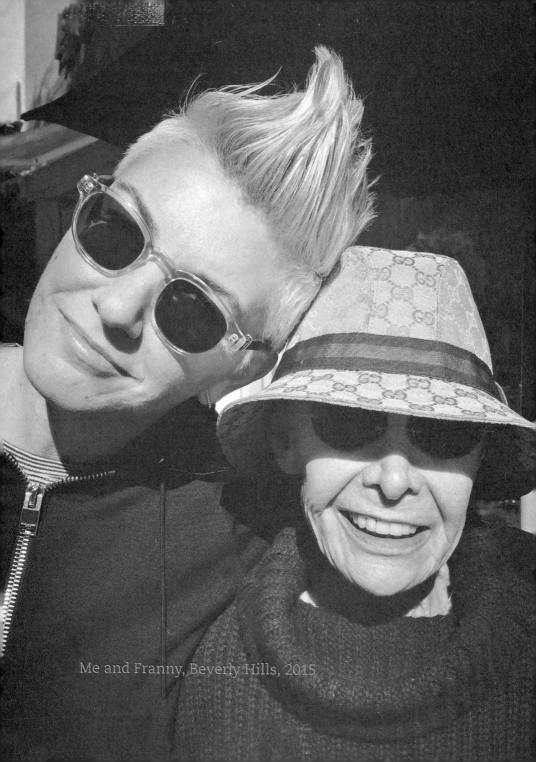

Me and Franny, Beverly Hills, 2015

## HOW EXERCISE AFFECTS YOUR BODY

"This is what exercise does for you," Dr. Steinbaum told me. "It dilates your arteries, which lowers your blood pressure. It lowers your bad cholesterol level and raises your good one. It keeps your blood sugar down. It releases serotonin, the feel-good brain chemical. It keeps your weight down. It gives you energy. And, of course, it keeps you young."

The best thing about exercise is that anyone can do it. If you have access to a gym or if you can attend classes, that's great, but it's not necessary because movement is movement and all of it is good. Walking is terrific exercise, especially when you walk *fast,* and walking is free. Knowing that you can walk your way to health means there are no excuses for not tying on your shoes!

Even better, you don't have to spend hours in the gym to begin reaping the health benefits of exercise. While as little as an hour a week—about nine minutes a day—will start to have an effect, according to the National Institute of Health, aiming for 150 minutes of moderate-intensity aerobic exercise each week is a key factor in reducing the risk of many chronic diseases. That's a mere two and a half hours a week. I know you can do that!

### How Exercise Affects Your Cardiorespiratory (Heart and Lung) Health

According to the American Heart Association, more than a third of American adults are at risk for cardiovascular disease. And while one in thirty-one American women dies from breast cancer every year, which is terrifying enough, one in three dies of heart disease. Hundreds of thousands of men and women die unnecessarily every year because of conditions they might have prevented—especially if they exercised.

The National Institutes of Health also make it clear how important exercise is, by stating, "The benefits of physical activity on cardiorespiratory health (affecting the heart, lungs, and blood vessels) are some of the most extensively documented of all the health benefits. . . . People who do moderate- or vigorous-intensity aerobic physical activity have a significantly lower risk of cardiovascular disease than do inactive people. Regularly active adults have lower rates of heart disease and stroke, and have lower blood pressure, better blood lipid profiles, and fitness."

One of the primary reasons for this is that your heart is a muscle, and all muscles respond to what's called overload. Yes, you can feel that being overloaded is a bad thing when too much is going on in your life, or when you pick up too many heavy boxes at the same time, but physical overload, within moderation, is a *good* thing. It's merely the physical stress your body undergoes when you're more active than usual. Your body is built to handle overload—it relishes it, actually, because this is how you get stronger. When you do any kind of aerobic activity, which increases your heart and breathing rate, your lungs need to work harder to get more oxygen to your muscles, and your heart has to pump harder to get more blood to those same muscles. Overload makes your entire cardiovascular system work more efficiently, and with more power. You'll be less prone to develop coronary heart disease. Your blood pressure should also decrease, which means less bad stress for the heart and a lower risk of stroke.

Exercise has also been proven to reduce LDL cholesterol (the bad type that leads to plaque forming in your arteries, clogging them and creating a higher risk of sudden heart attacks, strokes, and blood clots) while increasing HDL cholesterol (the good type that you need; cholesterol is a waxy substance your body must have to run your metabolism and hormone production properly). "In fact," Dr. Steinbaum told me, "HDL cholesterol is what protects your arteries, and the *only thing* you can do to raise its level is to exercise. You can't do it with food or medication." In addition, you have to watch your triglyceride levels; triglycerides are a fat component and part of the cholesterol package. They become elevated as a direct response to an unhealthy diet, especially one laden with sugars and simple carbohydrates. Often, those who tend to gain weight in their belly areas have dangerously high triglyceride levels—and what brings them down is exercise.

## How Exercise Affects the Rest of Your Body

Exercise doesn't just affect your cardiovascular system. Your entire body benefits.

Better bone and muscle strength. As we get older, our bones become more brittle and less dense, and our muscles will atrophy without regular use. Weight-bearing exercises that put stress on bones by means of impact or overload, such as running, Spinning, aerobics, dance, and weight training, help to strengthen them and improve density. The stronger your bones, the less likely you are to suffer from osteoporosis or debilitating fractures. The more you use your muscles, the stronger and more pliable they become. The fibers of the fascia, or the connective tissue surrounding your joints, are strengthened by exercise, keeping your joints flexible and less prone to injury.

Antiaging. As time goes by, gravity starts to pull you to the earth. I want to make sure that by the time that starts to happen, your body looks the best it's ever looked. The way to do that is to defy gravity by staying in motion. This means you want to build a lot of long, lean muscle in a nice long, lean way. You'll move better not just when you're young, but you'll remain strong as you grow older.

Exercise may also work on a cellular level to reverse the toll the aging process has on our bodies. According to a 2010 study from the University of California, San Francisco, for example, researchers found that stressed-out women who exercised vigorously for an average of forty-five minutes over a three-day period had cells that showed fewer signs of aging compared to women who were stressed and inactive.

The anti-inflammatory benefits of exercise also impact aging on a cellular level. What is inflammation? It's a normal, natural response to any kind of injury. But as we get older, our blood vessels get more inflamed, so they thicken. This affects blood transport to your cells, which need the nutrient-enriched blood to function properly. The more you exercise, the more your body can rid itself of protein molecules called cytokines, which act as a sort of molecular messenger to regulate your inflammatory response. (Too many cytokines can cause inflammatory diseases like rheumatoid arthritis, for example.)

And, of course, your skin always looks better when you exercise; not only do you get a rosy glow when your blood is pumping, but as science has told us, your skin is your body's largest organ. Take care of it, and it will take care of *you*.

Improved immune system. A strong and fit body is a body less likely to get sick and one that will recover more quickly from common illnesses like colds and the flu. Researchers at Appalachian State University in North Carolina found that people who exercised regularly were 23 percent less likely to get colds than those who exercised less.

Reduces likelihood of developing cancer. At least 35 percent of all cancer deaths may be related to obesity and lack of activity, the Seattle Cancer Research Center has found. And according to the National Cancer Institute, "Adults who increase their physical activity, either in intensity, duration, or frequency, can reduce their risk of developing colon cancer by 30 to 40 percent relative to those who are sedentary regardless of body mass index (BMI), with the greatest risk reduction seen among those who are most active."

I had a long discussion with Dr. Steinbaum about the biggest mistake people make when they work out, and although I don't see this in my classes, I do see it when I go to the gym. This is what she told me:

*The biggest mistake is that people don't actually know what "exercise" means. I had a patient one day who showed me her workout shoes. They were lovely sling-backs with kitten heels. I asked her where her sneakers were, and she told me she didn't own any. So I told her that whatever she was doing, it did not constitute exercise!*

*My patients often tell me that when they start to work out, they're short of breath, they're sweating, their hearts are pounding. They're scared that something's wrong. I always reassure them that nothing is wrong. That all those "symptoms" are what's supposed to happen when they exercise! That they're doing it right.*

*I can't tell you how many times I've heard that, and it's really a failure of education that people don't understand what aerobic exercise actually means and how much they need to do for optimum benefits. Based on recommendations of the American Heart Association, you should aim for 150 minutes each week of moderate aerobic exercise, and two days of strength training.*

*But here's where confusion sets in. Within those 150 minutes, your heart rate needs to be elevated. A simple stroll won't do that. A gentle ride on a recumbent bicycle at the gym won't do that. The easiest way to check how "moderate" your exercise is is to remember what it's like to answer a phone when it's ringing and you are breathing so hard you literally can't* quite speak in a complete sentence. If you can say a full sentence without pausing to catch your breath, you aren't working hard enough—you should aim for huffing and puffing.

Also, use a device on your wrist or on machines in the gym to monitor your heart rate. Your target heart rate (THR) should be 220 minus your age times 85 percent. (Remember to multiply the figure by .85, not 85!) You want to hit that number and sustain it for twenty minutes to get the maximum cardiovascular benefits of that exercise session. Don't go over your maximum heart rate. Stay just at or below it—not above!

In other words, you need to push yourself. If you do not get your heart rate up, you are not exercising right!

It's also extremely important to be mindful when you work out. If your mind is not engaged, your body isn't. Reading a magazine while you walk on a treadmill is not mindful exercise. Checking Instagram while you jog isn't mindful. Exercising isn't just about engaging your muscles—it's about engaging your entire body. Use this time wisely, and focus. When you do that, everything starts to change!

What a great doctor! Everything she says is just what I believe about setting intentions, mindfulness, and physical presence in your life. It's all about the *presence*, not the presents—you can buy all the gadgets you want, but nothing is going to bring you into reality more than being aware of what you're doing when you're exercising, and how well you're doing it.

THE BIGGEST MISTAKE PEOPLE MAKE ABOUT EXERCISE

The Institute also found that lower rates of breast and endo-metrial cancers could be linked to the exercise-triggered bene-fits of lower hormone production (for postmenopausal women) and weight management. Lung cancer rates also go down—how many smokers do you know who are regular exercisers?

Reduces type 2 diabetes and metabolic syndrome rates, espe-cially those related to obesity. Metabolic syndrome is a worrying health condition most people have never heard of—but they should, as it's often a signal that type 2 diabetes and/or heart disease is going to develop. It is characterized by having sev-eral medical conditions: high blood sugar, high blood pres-sure, excess weight (especially around the midsection), and abnormal cholesterol levels. Key to preventing it is a normal weight and regular exercise. Keeping your weight at normal levels also makes you far less likely to develop type 2 diabetes, which is an extremely serious and life-threatening disease. It's caused by insulin irregularities and an increasing inabil-ity to process nutrients due to blood sugar problems.

If you eat too many simple carbohydrates in the form of junk food, white flour and sugar, juice, and pasta, your body has a hard time processing it; your blood sugar spikes, a large amount of insulin is released by the pancreas to regulate it; and you are suddenly starving even if you've just eaten a large bagel. Worse, when you don't metabolize all the calories you eat, your body stores them . . . in the form of *fat*. That type 2 diabetes is on the rise is extremely alarming, especially when a good diet and exercise habits almost always prevent it from occurring.

Natural sleeping pill. The National Sleep Foundation has reported that those who exercise regularly not only have more energy during the day, but they sleep better at night. I can also tell you that exercise helps me nap, and I am a strong believer in the power nap. My short power naps keep me energized from morning till night, and I try to have one every day. I typically get my nap on after my morning classes and meetings. I allow for a minimum of twenty minutes, though sometimes I go for an hour, but no more, unless I'm sick, because then I try to sleep as much as I possibly can. The body completely recharges during sleep. I am convinced this is why I look twenty-nine at forty-eight. I sleep a *lot!*

## AOA = ADULT-ONSET ATHLETICISM

I work with students of many different ages, and lots of the adults want me to know right off the bat that they were never coordinated as kids, never got picked for teams at school, were never strong or athletic. It's their way of telling me not to expect much of them and letting me know that working out scares them. They've also got it in their heads that it's too late to train like an athlete.

I don't buy it—and here's what I tell them, courtesy of Bill Bowerman, cofounder of Nike: "If you have a body, you are an athlete."

Right away, I think of Geralyn, who came to me when she was a forty-five-year-old mom. Her last experience with team sports was sitting on the bench for her high school lacrosse team, and recently her only exercise was putting on Spanx, hopping on and off bar stools, and using a wineglass to do bicep curls. She was full of rage and full of frustration. She had no outlets for her stress. When we started working together, a memory flashed through her mind: "Will not pump on the playground swings."

"Ohmigod," she told me, through tears. "I was too scared to be strong. I couldn't even get on a *swing* at the local playground when I was a little girl."

I know it took a lot of courage to say she wanted to change. "And now look at you," I said. "You're *here*, right? It isn't going to take long at all for you to be in the best shape of your life. I'm going to show you that it didn't matter who you were—what matters is what you want to *become*."

I saw Geralyn in class at least three or four times a week. I saw that determined look on her face. I saw how she went from asking to be seated in the very back, on the bike farthest from the experienced riders—because she didn't want anyone looking at her and she was terrified she couldn't keep up the pace—to moving flat-out, at top speed, her dial turned firmly way past zero. Fast-forward six months, and Geralyn has lost twenty pounds. She breezes through my classes, which she still attends at least three or four times a week. She is buff and *strong*. She calls herself an athlete. She *is* an athlete.

Geralyn is proof that it is *never* too late to become an athlete. She's lucky because she's caught something I want everyone to have. I call it AOA—Adult-Onset Athleticism.

What is an athlete, after all? The dictionary says it's any person who is proficient in sports and other forms of physical exercise. A person who is trained or skilled in exercises, or in games requiring physical strength, agility, or stamina.

"It is never too late to become an athlete."

Got that? Did you see the words *team sports* anywhere in that? Of course not! As a society focused on team sports, we're conditioned to think of athletes as professionals who play on some kind of team and have coaches and have been training for years. If that's not you, it's really easy to count yourself out of the the realm of being an athlete. I'm here to tell you that's just wrong. You can embody your inner AOA in the way you regularly walk around your neighborhood with your dog.

AOA is all about changing how you see yourself and re-imagining your body's physical and emotional capabilities. AOA is about you discovering what kind of athlete you can be as a grown-up, especially if you were never nurtured as an athlete when you were a child. If that's you, you're in luck—I'm really sorry for how awful you might have felt when you were little, but you're my absolute favorite kind of adult to transform. Anyone who still has strong and damaging memories of always being the last one picked for any team during those dreaded gym classes, or who was the fat kid, or the clumsy kid, or the one who had a real fear of sports. Anyone who could never ride a bike or dive into a pool is the most rewarding student for those of us in the fitness industry.

I get a lot of new students who, like Geralyn, put themselves in the farthest corner in the back of the room. "I was never an athlete when I was younger," they tell me. "I'm so old now— look at me. I'm never going to get in shape. It's too late to start, isn't it? Did I miss my peak? I know I did. Forget it. I just want to get through this class."

This is what I tell them: "You're here. That's amazing. No way have you missed your peak. You are about to discover your *new* peak! So let's have some fun. Think of it as your moment to re-learn how to use your body, kick some ass, and once and for all feel good about participating in things that are physically good for you!"

I absolutely love watching my students blossom before my eyes. Often, it takes only a few weeks for me to see the beginnings of the transformation. That's an incredibly short period of time for someone who spent decades thinking they were never going to be strong or capable.

The reward comes as I get to watch the AOA come over them, like a spell being cast by a benevolent wizard. It happens because turning into an athlete isn't just about getting the muscles. It's about turning around that little voice in your head that says you're not one, that you're not coordinated and that you can't move. It's an amazing transformation, and it can happen to anyone.

If you're already comfortable calling yourself an athlete, this book is going to crank you up more than a few notches. If you're not an athlete, this book will turn you into one!

And you're going beyond just being a physical athlete—you're going to be an *emotional* athlete. That's actually far more important. You can't be a physical athlete without being an emotional athlete first. That means loving your body, setting goals and intentions, visualizing the future you want, taking some risks when you add more movement to your life, and believing in yourself.

And yes, it also means having the courage to walk through the door of a gym or a dance studio. There's risk—but good risk, the kind where you're challenging yourself to do something good, just for *you*. Because you need it. Because it's unbelievably good for you. And, most of all, because you *deserve* it!

Before I moved to New York, I used to go full-out during every class I taught, working out at least twelve hours every week. I don't do that anymore and couldn't even if I wanted to. I've had to have two arthroscopic surgeries and one major ACL reconstruction. I still walk around with two screws in my bones, one in my femur and one in my tibia. Does that stop me from finding something that works for me? No. I still train. Each week, I work out for myself at least twice, ride once or twice, and teach my twenty classes.

## Find Out What Kind of AOA Turns You On the Most

One of the best things about exercise is there's so much to choose from—so many completely wonderful ways to move. I have friends who love tennis and other racquet sports. They experience great joy from the mental acuity they develop while making split-second decisions about where to hit the ball, but they also find it deeply satisfying to *hit* a benign object for an hour or two.

Ditto with those who like to box (and believe me, you'll get killer arms, abs, and a butt like you won't believe if you box).

Some like the solitary pursuit of running because it gives them a chance to be alone with their thoughts and their music; I know a writer who plotted out an entire novel while she ran.

Some people crave the camaraderie you get from being on a team. Others just like to dance. I tell all my newbie AOAs to experiment with lots of different kinds of movement, and eventually you'll find something you really love. When you love it, it's going to be much easier to stick to it.

If you like a particular sport or kind of exercise but you feel like something is missing, you can be creative and make up your own version. When my dad was going through treatment for stage IV bladder cancer, to help him get through such a stressful and debilitating time, he came up with his own version of Tai Chi. He had always had his own version of stretching out slowly, and did it every day, so I'm not sure it was even a "type" of Tai Chi, but it was his . . . and he was into it, so it worked for him up until the end.

When I was determined to keep myself away from my old unhealthy lifestyle, I decided the only way I could heal myself was through exercise. But I took a very important lesson from my dad's slowly-stretching-out-every-day routine when I also decided I needed a kind of exercise I'd never done before. I knew if I took on something that ended up being too easy for me physically, I would become bored and that could cause me to slip back into old bad habits I didn't want to do.

I decided I would take up yoga, and to get started I signed on to do a two-month course in Mysore, India. This was not New York trendy yoga—it was Sri K. Patthabhi Jois Ashtanga yoga, the real deal.

In Mysore, I stayed with my friend Kelly in a beautiful little house. I found the course incredibly therapeutic, but at the same time, I realized real-deal Ashtanga yoga was not for me. I need loud music and fast movement to stay committed—that's just how I'm hardwired. But there was no way I was going to quit my stint there because it was such an incredible adventure, and because I had made my mind up to stick out what I had committed to do.

So while I was doing my yoga poses for hours every day and still reaping its rewards and becoming more flexible than I ever thought possible, I kept coming up with all these ideas of how to improve the yoga experience for *me*.

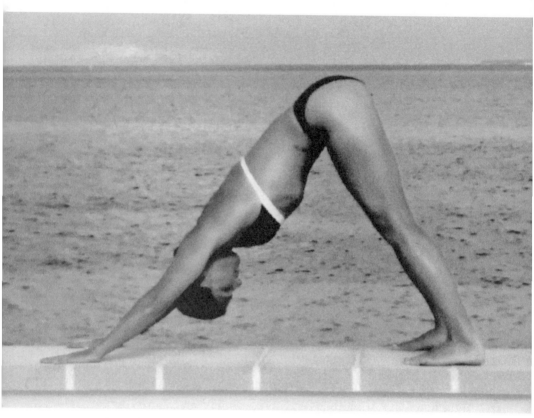

After three months of study in India, 2001

I suddenly realized one day that I wasn't just going to teach yoga—I was going to adapt the best principles of yoga (being present, focus on breathing, learning stillness, visualizations, meditations, using your own body strength without any props, core strength, flexibility) and put them to music and create my own workout system.

I wouldn't ever dream of calling it yoga, because the yogis would have been appalled—and after all, it *wasn't* real yoga! But it was the kind of exercise and mindfulness I knew I liked, and I liked it because it worked for *me*. I also figured my students would like the more dynamic aspects of it, too.

At the same time, with exercise giving me the physical rush and emotional discipline that were healing everything I was suffering from, there was no way I was going to stop doing it. So that was my way of turning my own knob way past zero—and that is what's brought me to the place of calm and peace and accomplishment as a teacher I never thought I'd find.

## Visualization—Motivation for Any Workout

Use this visualization when you find yourself asking why you should even bother working out. You know *why* you should, but sometimes your brain takes over from your body. You know that getting a move on isn't just about physicality—it's about finding the mental focus and feeling it in your heart. In this moment, I would use a song you love with a strong beat that will help you focus while you visualize. Also, read how to do it first, then put the book down, the song on, and give it a shot!

Note: This visualization technique will *only* work if you back it up with the action that will actually take you there. Here's what I mean by this: If your meditation is about having flatter abs, don't think about lunch—think about dropping on the floor and doing the planks or the sit-ups *after* you do the meditation.

This is the trick to putting the meditation to actual work; see it *first* in your head . . . then go friggin' do it! You have to *truly believe* in what you see in your mind. When you start doubting, you unwind the process. . . . *Do not doubt! Then get into action!*

1. Close your eyes and picture yourself in your absolute favorite destination, looking the way you've always wanted to look. You have to create a genuine focus on what you're about to do and how you plan to do it. You can't stop thinking about what you want to look like, because if your mind drifts, you start thinking about other things. As you think, breathe . . . deeply, and with each breath, feel the changes as if they are showing up every time you inhale and exhale.

2. Continue to see yourself down to the clothes you're wearing, the way you feel in them, and the shoes on your feet. Be strong. Imagine your body changing into exactly what you've always wanted it to be. Everything about you is changing. Every day it's changing for the better. *What is that?* you ask. That's mind, body, soul. That's what makes you want to cry! You imagining yourself as a better version of you should bring tears to your eyes. Being in shape and having the body you want is an emotional and physical labor of love.

3. The key to putting this all together is finding the workouts, the movements, the rituals of exercise to get you in motion and keep you in motion. As you continue to visualize yourself, think about what it is that makes you happy and ex-

cited when you do it—this could be running, speed walking, swimming, indoor cycling, tennis, whatever . . .

After your visualization, your next step is making the right time to bring motion into your life, as well as finding a teacher to give you instruction for your sport or activity. We live in a wonderful Internet age of Google and other search engines where you can get a lot of information. Try out a few different instructors to see who suits your personality. Sometimes it takes a while to find the perfect fit. Be patient and have fun while you're looking!

## DON'T LET FEAR HOLD YOU BACK

Not long ago, a woman named Denise came up to me before class started and said, "I have to let you know that I might not be able to do the push-ups today because I had a mastectomy." I thanked her for telling me and asked her how long ago she'd had it. She told me it had been a year. Wait a minute—a *year?*

"Come with me," I told Denise as I took her out to a quiet corner in the hallway. "Okay, tell me, if you can, what's really going on. You've had a year to heal, which should be long enough for you, physically, at least. Is that true?"

She nodded, so I went on. "So I need you to let go of that mentally," I added. "Let go of your diagnosis. Let go of your

# PLAYLIST
## FOR AOA

These songs will help you get into the groove, and stay there.

| | |
|---|---|
| Aerosmith | "Sweet Emotion" |
| Toni Braxton | "You're Making Me High" |
| Coldplay | "Hymn for the Weekend" |
| DNCE | "Cake by the Ocean" |
| Kirk Franklin | "Brighter Day" |
| FUTURPOETS | "Superman" |
| David Guetta | "Lift Me Up (Mylo Mix)" |
| George Michael | "Faith" (Aeroplane Remix) |
| Bruno Mars | "24K Magic" |
| Justin Timberlake | "Can't Stop the Feelin'" |

mastectomy. Let go of everything that happened. Don't let that be what's identifying how and who you are. This is a new you. Letting go of what happened last year is the best thing you can do right now. We're going to rebuild you in every possible way, and you're going to be the strongest student in my class today. Do the push-ups today and don't be afraid to do them the best way you can. If you feel any discomfort at all from the scar tissue, then please listen to your body and go easy. It doesn't matter if your form isn't perfect or if you can't go all the way down and up. Don't even think about that. I know you can do it."

Her eyes filled with tears that she quickly blinked away.

"You're still here, and you need to kick ass," I added. "So let's freaking kick ass today!"

"Thank you, Stacey," she said as she turned to go back inside.

I kept a careful eye on her during class, and when we got to the push-ups I saw she *was* doing them. And doing them really well, I might add. That's when I moved near her and gave her a big smile and a thumbs-up.

When the class was over, I stood by the door as I always do to fist-bump my students as they leave, giving them the acknowledgment they deserve for their hard work. Denise smiled when she saw me.

"That was the best advice *ever*," she said. "You really got me through it."

"I'm glad," I replied. "I knew you weren't going to hurt yourself. You're *strong* now. You're *so much* stronger than you think."

Denise had finally allowed herself to push past the fear. Her muscles were sturdy; her brain was not. She was still thinking of herself as a victim rather than a warrior who'd fought the enemy that had tried to kill her—and vanquished it.

The new determination on Denise's face made me think of another one of my longtime students, Maria Pargac, whom I told you about on page 174. Her late-stage breast cancer had spread to some of her lymph nodes. Her oncologist told her it wasn't looking good, that it was likely terminal. During surgery, most of her pectoral muscle was removed, and she was told that due to the trauma, she'd never have muscles there again.

Maria was determined to get better, and she asked me for help. When we would focus before class, I would tell her to visualize her pec muscles coming back, to see herself as whole and strong again. Well, you should see Maria's pec muscles now from doing all the push-ups in class—muscles her doctors were sure would be gone for good. I would love to see the look on those doctors' faces now when she goes in for her checkups! She is beyond buff. I am in awe of her guts and determination.

The difference between Denise and Maria was stark. Maria told herself on day one of her diagnosis that she was a general in the army of her life, and she was going to defeat the enemy, whatever the doctors said. Her disease actually empowered her. She fired up her mental cancer carpet duster, and she started using it to beat that old rug to get all the entrenched dirt and grime out until she won.

Denise took a different approach. She, too, was a general, but it took her much longer to fight the battle. She had a lot more fear to conquer. Finally, it was power she got from exercise that gave her the last bit of courage she needed. Denise needed me to tell her it was okay to be fierce—and *to freaking kick ass*.

## Time to Shed the Excuses

I've been working as a fitness professional for so long I could swear I've heard every possible excuse a person could come up with to skip their workouts. Here's a list of some of them, matched up with what you can tell yourself when one goes through your mind.

| No, I Can't | Oh Yes, You Can |
| --- | --- |
| I don't have the time. | You have time to shop, to prepare your meals, to go get your hair done for special occasions. You spend time taking care of your kids, and now it is time to take care of yourself. |
| A gym membership is too expensive. | Exercise is free. Walking is one of the best exercises for you, and it doesn't cost anything. Working out to exercise shows on TV or via streaming is free. (There are lots of incredible workouts on YouTube, and they're all free!) In addition, what else are you spending money on that you can cut down on or eliminate? |
| I'm afraid to use the equipment in the gym. | It's always a good idea to hire a professional personal trainer for a session or two when you go to a gym—they'll show you the right way to work out for your body. This will not only prevent injuries but improve your workouts right away. Many people get hurt because they don't know the right way to use weights or equipment and are too shy to ask. Speak up. Ask for help! You're paying to be there! |
| I don't have space in the house. | You can leave the house and take a walk. |
| I don't have the right gear. | You can wear anything comfortable to exercise. Think of what cavemen wore to do it. There's no reason to spend a lot of money on designer clothes that you're going to sweat in, right? |
| I just had surgery, and I'm sore. | Discuss when you can start a modified program with your surgeon and/or physical therapist. Start slow and listen to your body. *(cont.)* |

| No, I Can't | Oh Yes, You Can *(cont.)* |
|---|---|
| I have exercise-induced asthma. | See a pulmonologist. An inhaler might help a lot. Exercise can actually improve lung function, but be sure not to overdo it. (Asthma is no joke. Always, *always* consult your doctor before you do any kind of exercise.) |
| I have an injury. | All athletes get injured at some point—it goes with the territory. They rest and heal until they're given the go-ahead to start working out again, and then they're right back at it. |
| Everyone is going to make fun of me. | If anyone is so shallow as to judge another person's body or abilities, they're losers who aren't worth thinking about. Besides, people are almost always much more concerned with their own workouts than they are with looking at or thinking about anyone else at the gym or anywhere else. |

I do understand why these excuses are said. Finding time *can* be hard. Going from inactive to active *is* hard. Feeling that you're being judged (even if you're not) *is* a valid fear—walking into any new gym or studio can be daunting, even for experienced exercisers. Learning how to do any new sport or dance moves or exercises *is* sometimes really tough. Especially if doing so came much more easily to you when you were younger. As we get older, flexibility or stamina don't come as easily anymore. You can also be experiencing a painful twinge of ruefulness about your own mortality. But are you going to wallow in it? Of course not! You're going to get up and kick ass today!

So when I hear any of these excuses, I always walk my students through whatever it is they're saying, and together we find solutions. There's *always* a solution.

Especially when it comes to the time factor. Most people think exercise must be done in chunks of at least thirty minutes, but that's not true. A study done at McMaster University in Hamilton, Ontario, with results published in 2016, found that you can reap the benefits of just one minute of intense exercise each day—not that you should do so little, but your body instantly responds.

There have been other, numerous studies showing that those who split their exercise time into ten-minute increments were more likely to exercise consistently. In one study, women who divided up their exercise sessions lost more weight after five months than women who exercised for twenty to forty minutes at a time.

In a landmark study conducted at the University of Virginia, exercise physiologist Glenn Gaesser, PhD, asked men and women to complete fifteen 10-minute exercise routines a week. After just twenty-one days, the volunteers' aerobic fitness was equal to that of people ten to fifteen years younger. "It would be useful for people to get out of the all-or-nothing mind-set that unless they exercise for thirty minutes, they're wasting their time," he said.

I saw this myself in 2007 when I worked on a program called Healthy Upgrade Team with Brooke Shields for Colgate, an ad campaign targeting women to help them take better care of their teeth. My part of the process was to challenge women to get moving. I came up with a regime that had them scrubbing pots in a circular pattern, brushing their teeth with extra oomph, mopping the floor with their feet—you get the idea. The women we worked with didn't equate cleaning with exercise until we showed them how pushing a heavy vacuum back and forth did wonders for their arms and butts.

It makes sense; when you're actively cleaning, your body is in motion. You just need to take the time to focus on the kinesiology of how you're actually using your muscles, instead of just performing the task. You will be surprised how sore you can get from mopping the floor with your feet!

I know it is more challenging today to be active than in previous generations. As unfathomable as it might seem to anyone born after 1970, back in the day, people actually had to get up to answer the telephone and change the TV channels; they even had to wash all the dishes by hand.

Decades ago, kids walked or biked to school. Now there are buses and carpools. These same kids would come home from school and then go out to play. Now helicopter parents are too scared not to have a GPS blinking on their little ones' cell phones.

If you had to research a project, you'd go to a library and stand in front of the card catalogue and then walk around the shelves and reach up and down for the books you needed. Now all you have to do is hit the search button on your browser. Sed-

You can do this either sitting or standing. This sequence is surprisingly tough, especially when you keep a lot of tension on the shirt (or you can use a towel). For a harder workout, you can repeat this up to one hundred times if you want to go crazy! Knock yourself out.

1. Grab a T-shirt and hold it with one hand at each end.

2. Position your hands at 9 and 3 on the clock and move the T-shirt from side to side for 5 seconds.

3. Move your hands to 12 and 6 on the clock. Hold the hand at 12 steady while circling the hand at 6 as if you are stirring a pot of thick oatmeal.

4. Move your hands to do a bicep curl, and then when your hands are at shoulder height, extend them upward, over your head. Do as many as you can for 10 seconds.

5. Move your left hand to forehead height, palm facing out, and your right hand in the bicep curl position. Move the T-shirt up and down on a diagonal for 5 seconds. Switch sides and repeat. Do not overextend the upper arm too much—it's not about moving the T-shirt too high but about feeling the tension in your triceps.

THE THIRTY-SECOND
T-SHIRT WORKOUT

entary jobs have increased 83 percent since 1950; physically active jobs now make up less than 20 percent of our workforce, compared to 1960, when about half of the US workforce was physically active.

The consequences and problems from lack of movement are deadly. In all, sedentary lifestyles lead to an estimated 5.3 million premature deaths a year worldwide, right up there with smoking.

Half an hour of brisk walking every day can do more for your long-term health than all the efforts of a dozen doctors and their medication. (The key word is *brisk,* as you need to get your heart pumping, as Dr. Steinbaum explained on page 272.) Thirty minutes is all you need—whether from walking, jogging, running, using machines at the gym, biking, dancing, or swimming. Every day.

I don't care how you move, but I want you to get up and get a move on. Even just doing a minute or two is a start. Rosanna Scotto is the cohost of a local morning TV show, *Good Day New York,* and she asked me to come on the program one day to reach those viewers sitting on the couch who didn't have exercise equipment like an indoor bike at their disposal. I wanted to reach the viewers who knew they should be exercising, but still weren't.

Together, Rosanna and I decided to demonstrate a thirty-second T-shirt workout that anyone can find the time to do. (It was all the time they had in the segment for us to do the moves!) We hoped it would trigger these people to see how easily they could incorporate a really fun little sequence of movement into their lives, even while they were watching TV.

Obviously, you *can't* change your body in thirty seconds, but you can trigger some endorphins, capture a small amount of motivation, and possibly activate your brain to challenge yourself and do something bigger as a result of the thirty-second kick-start!

It *is* easy, and it *is* fun. Gradually, I want your magic number to increase so you're aiming for 150 minutes of movement a week. Or more!

## Finally Confronting Fear Itself

I'm pretty fearless, but even I have my moments. I know the primary reason people don't do the things they dream of—whether it's starting a new business, moving, opening their heart to love, standing up to a bully, treating themselves with the nurturing care they deserve and making better eating and working out habits a regular part of their lives—is fear.

Fear of the unknown, fear of rejection, fear of failure.

When I got the call that I was going out with Oprah Winfrey on her "Life You Want" tour in November 2014, I had to sit down for a minute. I was told I'd be training fifteen thousand people. All at once. You gotta give me this one. Yes, I, the fearless Stacey, had a moment of sheer, blind panic.

*No way,* I told myself, *that fifteen thousand people are going to get up out of their seat and do this workout. No freaking way! What if they don't like my teaching? What if I ask them to get up, and they stay in their seats? What if, what if, what if?*

Was I listening to my own normal, confident self? Nope. That blind moment of sheer panic took residence in my brain the entire time I was working with Angela Davis, who was teaching Sheri Salata (president of Harpo Productions) and Oprah at SoulCycle at the time. She lived in Los Angeles, and I was in New York, so we had to create the routine over Skype, using a two-by-two-foot space because we knew the partici-

I had horrible posture as a kid. It was so bad that my dad would make me stand against a wall with a book on my head to practice what it was like to keep my shoulders back! My mom would also constantly say, "Stand up straight!"

They knew that posture is important. It speaks volumes about you because the second you walk through the door, it's the first thing anybody sees. You always want to walk into any room with your head up and your eyes focused on some point in the distance to elongate your neck—as if you were clad in an enormous velvet cloak, and you were dragging it regally behind you.

Pattabhi Jois, the founder of Ashtanga or "flow" yoga, was a teacher famous for the head-up-high/cloak-behind-you method of thinking. He is the reason Ashtanga became what it is today.

And this means, of course, that you are not looking down at the cell phone glued to your hand. Doing this is terrible for your posture,

pants were going to be in a stadium, in their seats, not on bikes, and we had to keep the movements small so they wouldn't be whacking the people sitting next to them. It took us about two months to figure it out, and I spent the entire time working myself into a tizzy.

*What if they don't like what we're doing?* I asked myself. *There's just no way this is going to work. I mean, Oprah's people, most of* especially the muscles of your neck and upper back. It's also terrible for your ability to open your eyes and see what's truly happening around you.

When you show up in the morning with your intentions set and a positive attitude, good vibrations are going to start passing through your body automatically. Remember, thoughts *are* vibrating inside you, so keep them positive. Pass the negative ones like clouds; just let them leave your head. It's the positive ones that you have on repeat . . . those are the ones that vibrate through you and keep your disposition on point. They're going to give you energy. They're going to make you push past your fears. They're going to make stride wherever it is you're going with power and confidence.

I still battle the rolled-shoulder syndrome thanks to all my years of riding the bike, and I have to really think about it when I go anywhere. You need to pay more attention, too. That, and keeping your chin from jutting out and leading your gait with your head sticking out. Try it. It works!

STAND TALL—IT WORKS

*them are women, are going to be in nice clothes because Oprah asked them to be in their Sunday best, and a lot of them won't be in fantastic shape. Nobody's going to want to do it right after lunch; they'll be tired. I'm going to make a total fool out of myself and Oprah is going to think I suck. Of all the people on this planet I want to impress, at the top of my list is* Oprah . . . *and I'm in a complete self-doubt zone!*

Finally, the big day arrived, and I showed up at the Prudential Center in New Jersey with my Soul army in tow. There were twelve people onstage on bikes, and me in front of them cueing the "#soul-15" workout Angela and I created. As soon as I started talking and showing the crowd what to do, sure enough, every single person was jumping up and down in their Sunday best, enjoying the movements we'd devised—and having a blast.

They easily followed our lead, watching us and repeating everything I showed them. I could tell, because they'd been given light-up wristbands. Every single light was moving in unison, all thirty thousand arms, like a magical army of fire-flies. (You can see snippets of it on YouTube at www.youtube .com/results?search_query=oprah+live+the+life+you+want +tour+soul+cycle.)

All my fears melted away, and I was filled with a pure surge of ecstatic energy, watching those wonderful participants as they shouted out wild whoops of joy and power. It was one of my proudest moments as a teacher.

Afterward, when the adrenaline was finally melting away, I had to have a tough conversation with myself. It was one of my biggest life lessons *ever*. I had allowed myself to become so fearful, and I had to push past the fear. I had to learn that I could not torture myself by being too scared to try. Never again.

After all, what was the worst thing that could have happened to me that day? I could have missed that opportunity by passing on it altogether. I could have said no just because the thought of fucking up in front of fifteen thousand people was so unbelievably terrifying!

Actually, once we got to Seattle, I did get caught up in a wardrobe malfunction, but at that point I had already done two cities, and I knew the audiences. I still remember seeing people up in the rafters dancing and jumping, and they were so far away their heads were the size of pins.

I often think of that day when a new student comes up to me before class and tells me he or she is scared, that everyone else knows what they're doing, and that they won't be able to do it. "Nobody else in the class matters except you," I always tell them. "You have your own bike; you have your own seat; you have your own space. And in my class nobody's looking at anybody else. No one cares."

You know why no one cares?

Two reasons. One, they are concentrating so hard on what they're doing that they don't see anyone else. And two, it starts at the top. It starts with who's creating the vibe in the room. And my vibe is focused on each and every person who's there to work. They are setting their intentions. That's more than enough to deal with!

"Besides," I go on, "you have your own will, and you have your own goals. So you don't have to worry about anything. It's not like we're in a boat and you have an oar and you go the wrong way and your oar's going to hit theirs and the boat is going to topple over and sink. That's not why we're here. You're going to be in your own universe in this studio, inside of a bigger universe. You're going to turn that knob past zero, and you're going to have the ride of your life."

## Moving Meditation—Motivation to Push Past the Fear

If the fear is getting to you, this Moving Meditation ought to help. As you need to keep your eyes closed, do this one when you are moving on a stable piece of equipment, such as a Spin bike, a recumbent bicycle, or a rowing machine. You can also do it when holding on to the edge of a pool and kicking, or marching in place in your home.

1. Close your eyes and see yourself in your mind's eye. You are a vivacious, strong human being. There is a reason why you were born a human being and not a book or a tree. You were meant to do special and amazing things.

2. Picture yourself climbing or cycling up a hill. I don't know what's at the top of the hill. Only *you* know. This is only about *you* and your goals—not anyone else's. The top of this hill is you pushing as hard as you possibly can against resistance. That's what the top of the hill means in real life. You are climbing your personal mountain. This is your hill, baby. This is your time. This is your place. This is your workout. This moment belongs to you.

3. Keep climbing until you get to the top. That's where you'll

# PLAYLIST
## FOR WORKING OUT

Even if I'm having a draggy kind of day, when I walk into the studio, where seventy expectant faces are turned toward me, I know there's one easy thing guaranteed to get me in the mood: I turn the music up. *Way* up. And then I am ready to kick butt. It *never* fails!

These particular songs are relatable to the same vibration that makes you want to instantly get up and get on the dance floor. They're some of my favorites that are all extremely propulsive in feeling, with that sexy beat that literally compels you to move.

| | |
|---|---|
| Astor | "Flashback" |
| Michael Chiklis/David Bowie | "The Way to Dirty Fame" |
| Depeche Mode | "Policy of Truth" |
| Dirty Vegas | "Tonight" |
| deadmau5 | "Let Go" |
| Demi Lovato | "Old Ways" |
| Pink | "Fuckin' Perfect" |
| Lisa Shaw | "Like I Want To" |
| Taylor Swift | "Better than Revenge" |
| Yelawolf | "Till It's Gone By" |

find what you want: your goals, your dream job, your next big project, more goals, more dreams, your love.

4. Instantly, you are flooded with an indescribable sensation of accomplishment and happiness, and you stand there for a minute, basking in the love.

5. You hear a soft, sweet, but determined voice saying, *Let it all out. Let out everything you've got through your breath. . . . Celebration, frustration, happiness, anxiety, anticipation, fear—all of it, let it out, exhale it out. Every emotion you ever had, let it out. You cannot keep it all inside. You have got to let it out in your life. This is your safe place. This is where the hot air comes out of your body, and the courage and strength is breathed in as you inhale.*

6. Take another deep breath. You let it all out. You are in charge.

7. Slowly, you imagine yourself living *inside* the goals you just visualized. You see that you are several thoughts away from actually manifesting these things into your life.

Now it's time to leave the Moving Meditation and go put these awesome thoughts into physical action. Go send the e-mail, send the text, make the phone calls to the people who can help you bring your visualization into reality. Do it *now!*

This will change the trajectory of your life. If you can do these visualizations during exercise, while you're in motion, you will have a bigger chance that they may actually come true, especially if, after the meditation, you actually *put them in motion!*

I know how well these visualizations work, because I've been told they do, hundreds of times over the last two decades, from the people who actually do this regularly.

You can be one of them!

So mark this page, put this book down, and send a text or e-mail that puts one of your goals or dreams in motion!

## HOW EXERCISE AFFECTS YOUR BRAIN

Did your professors at college lectures or the speakers at a TED Talk or an online seminar sit at a desk or in a chair? No—they are always in motion. They're walking back and forth. They're waving their hands and writing on SMART Boards. They're not doing this just so they can make eye contact with everybody in the audience.

They're doing it instinctively because their brains need them to move so they can get their message across most effectively. And they do this because movement stimulates brain activity, emotionally and intellectually. So if you want a brain boost, get up and get going. Anything that's good for your heart is going to be good for your brain, too—more blood flow means more thinking power.

Still not sure? Well, Dr. John Ratey, author of *Spark: The Revolutionary New Science of Exercise and the Brain,* says, "Exercise is the single best thing you can do for your brain in terms of mood, memory, and learning. Even ten minutes of activity changes your brain."

Scientists used to think the brain stopped growing when we were around age four, but fortunately we now know that just isn't true. Your brain cells, or neurons, are constantly being formed, even when you're past the age of retirement. This is called neuroplasticity or neurogenesis.

"All new learning creates new synapses in your brain," Michael Gonzalez-Wallace, a professional trainer and author of

*Super Body Super Brain,* a mind/body exercise system particularly designed to stimulate brain activity, told me after class one day.

"We use the word *plastic* to show how adaptable to change and stimulus your brain is. The more complicated the movements you do are—even if they're actually very simple, what counts is to have your brain *think* they're complicated—the more brain activity you'll stimulate."

This is why one of my favorite reasons to exercise is brain growth. In the same way that learning a new language long after you're out of school wakes up a dormant part of your brain, exercise stimulates the release of growth factors called brain-derived neurotropic factor (BDNF) that increase neurogenesis. BDNF is what allows your brain to grow new connections between neurons—and the more connections we can form, the better "shape" our brains are in. This is an extremely important factor in keeping your memory strong—especially as exercise stimulates activity in the temporal lobe, which is responsible for storing sensory memories—and to help prevent degenerative brain diseases like Alzheimer's disease.

For even more brain power, try doing exercises or a sport that constantly challenge your *thinking* as well as your moving; any kind of dance, for example, where you have to learn new sequences and remember steps, is a fantastic brain stimulator. So are racquet sports, where you're always trying to think of *where* to hit the ball even as you're hitting it. Mixing it up is always a good idea. Intersperse your runs or lap swimming or machines at the gym with a Zumba or yoga class. Your body will thank you. So will your brain.

## Your Very Own Dr. Feel-Good: How Exercise Helps Regulate Your Emotions

Every time you move or work out, you stimulate neurotransmitters, signaling nerve cells in your brain to fire up and get a move on. Your heart rate rises, your body temperature rises, your metabolism kicks in, and you got it poppin'. Your brain is on chemical fire. This is how you change your attitude in life. You simply move, and your brain does the rest.

The most important neurotransmitters for movement are serotonin, dopamine, norepinephrine, and endorphins. Serotonin is linked to muscle stimulation, memory, moods, digestion, and sleep. Dopamine and norepinephrine regulate movement, but they also deal with emotional responses.

Endorphins are truly unique. They are released when you exercise, and not only do they help us regulate pain and stress, but they can induce a glowing feeling of euphoria. You feel a rush of sweet happiness, and while you're feeling so good, these endorphins are also improving your immune and circulatory systems while they reduce stress and improve memory.

Much better than just a cup of coffee to get you going, right?

Endorphins and other brain chemicals are released and stimulated during exercise, and this can help to regulate your moods. In some cases, this can act as a natural antidepressant—

without the side effects of prescription medications. My father is a perfect example of this. Let me tell you why. . . .

My dad was diagnosed with bladder cancer in 2014, when he was seventy-two years old. He had been healthy and was taking care of himself and eating well and was always active for his entire life. He was an avid sportsman and was especially good at tennis, golf, and bowling. It was this athletic attitude that made him able to fight his cancer for as long as he did.

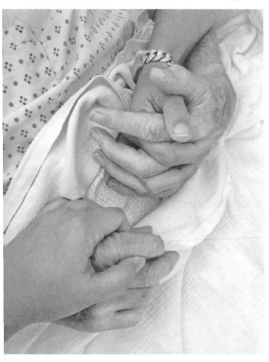

Me, Tiff, and Poppa

From the minute of his diagnosis, he had a difficult cancer to treat. His bladder was removed and replaced with an artificial one; it was often very painful and uncomfortable. But this is what he said to his oncologists: "I don't care what the plan is—whatever you say to do, I'm gonna do it. Radiation, chemotherapy, you just tell me what I have to do. As long as I can still play golf. I need to make sure I'm okay to get out on the course."

My dad had a true warrior spirit. He refused to sit at home and give up. He went to the hospital, had his chemo and radiation treatments, and then went straight to the course to play golf.

I was so proud of my dad's attitude, up until the day he died more than two years after a dire diagnosis. He didn't complain. He was very realistic. He adjusted to his illness; he needed to take more frequent naps, and sometimes he lost his appetite and my stepmom had to nag him to eat. For the most part, his attitude was amazing. I was in awe of his courage.

Given the circumstances, my dad had every right to be depressed about his diagnosis and treatment. Anyone who has cancer does. (Anyone who has any kind of difficult circumstances can develop depression or anxiety, and justifiably so.) But he absolutely did not let himself get depressed. He never saw himself as a victim. He rarely even talked about it—more to protect his family than anything else, I think.

Part of what kept my dad going was that he was always a very personable man, and he loved people. He had a great relationship with all of his doctors at the VA Hospital at Stanford University. He passed that attitude down to all of us in the family. So his attitude kept him going through the pain. His general love for life was his elixir.

So was physical activity. Sports were an active component of my dad's healing. He played golf up until a few months before his death. The fact that my dad was so fit absolutely helped him not be as sick as somebody his age who's overweight or a smoker. If he'd been out of shape and had not taken care of himself his entire life, we would have lost him much sooner. It's not so much that optimal health is a guarantee of letting you live a long life (although of course, it's an essential component)—it's that when something bad happens, being healthy gives you the stamina to help you heal quicker.

In addition, my dad had always done his own version of Tai Chi. As long as I can remember, I have memories of him doing his routine for about ten minutes every day. There's no name for it; it was just his own thing. He didn't study Tai Chi—he made it all up! He'd stretch, touch his toes, put his hands in a salutation, move around his head, balance or center himself, in a sequence he figured out on his own. He was amazingly flexible. He was my superstar.

I see my dad as a shining example of how to use your brain to power through trauma. After a daunting and terrifying delivery of bad news, he took the bull by the horns and went for it. He could have given up and watched TV all day while eating ice cream on the sofa and feeling sorry for himself. He definitely needed that ice cream to keep his weight up, but he went out there golfing and living his life instead of staying home in bed. If he'd given up, he would have died very quickly.

Not only did exercise keep my dad going up until the end, it helped him manage his stress. Whenever something stresses us in a good way (like getting a huge, challenging new project at work) or a bad way (the rent's going up and you just lost your job; your children are having a hard time at school; your car engine just gave out for the last time), your body instinctively releases the corticosteroid hormones cortisol and epinephrine. These hormones give you a noticeable jolt of energy that can help you make effective snap decisions, such as swerving out of the way of a drunk driver when you're on the road.

But if you're under prolonged stress, the continual release of these hormones can wreak havoc on your body, leaving you with such problems as irritability, sleep disorders, anxiety, and depression. In other words, your stress makes your stress more stressful.

As much as my dad was able to manage his stress, he knew what was happening to his body. We were always sanguine about his prospects. He had a goal. He wanted to see my nephew graduate from high school, and I was heartbroken, along with the rest of my family, that he wasn't able to make it. He was determined not to die *from* bladder cancer—he told himself he was going to die *with* it—and he was going to golf his way out of this life on his own terms. He fought up till the very end, and lived much longer than his doctors expected he would.

You might not be able to put an end to stressful situations that are out of your control (your parents getting a surprise divorce, for example, or a close friend becoming seriously ill), but you can do your utmost to manage them with specific techniques, such as mindful breathing, meditation, yoga, the kind of visualizations you've learned how to do in this book, and, of course, exercise. It's such a great stress reliever because the endorphins that are released during exercise automatically lower your cortisol levels. Not only will you feel better while you're moving—

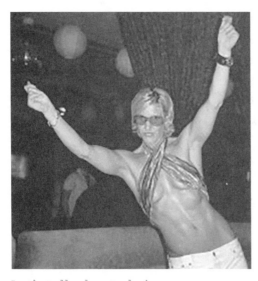

Let's talk about abs!

you'll continue to feel better *after* your workout is over.

Using exercise for regular stress management will not only help keep you on an even keel, it will improve your confidence and motivation.

I want to be clear that exercise can't *cure* depression, anxiety, or other mental illnesses. When things go wrong and you're having a particularly difficult time, you need to get the right kind of help—from a therapist, sometimes from medications, and especially from things you can do yourself that are guaranteed to make you feel better. Exercise will always be at the top of that list.

But making your physical fitness a priority will help you maintain a balance to face difficult moments so you don't trip and fall when you need to look calm, cool, and collected. This can happen when you need to be strong and go straight through a door to a meeting where you have to give a presentation and your nerves usually get the better of you. You know what I'm talking about, right?

We all have those days . . . we all have those moments . . . it doesn't matter who you are or what you have or what you've already done, we will all have those moments when you just have to have your shit together and do what you have to do.

You can either falter, or you can get *moving*—you know this in your body memory from the feeling you get from movement and exercise that you *can do this,* and you take that same memory and apply it to what you need to unleash the cascade of chemicals in your brain, enabling the gears to start turning so that you'll get the confidence and ideas and motivation and lift off you need.

You'll turn into a rocket that blasts off so you can do your thing, the way *you* want to do it. And succeed the way *you* want to.

## MY FAVORITE EXERCISES TO HELP YOU GET STACEY ABS

When you're getting fit and losing weight, you naturally think about your belly and what goes into it. These abs exercises are a perfect reinforcement for your core—the seat of all your physical strength and power.

When I was in my twenties and started training clients at my local gym, one of my best classes was my abs class. I always had great abs from playing sports, and fine-tuned the routine I taught based on what I'd learned from my swim coach and basketball coach in high school. They'd drilled into us that core strength is the root of all body strength, and that if you didn't have an awesome core, you wouldn't ever be a good athlete. I just had to look at my winning teammates for proof: Their abs were *ripped!*

The average American spends approximately fifty-six hours per week sitting, so their core automatically weakens. Add in improper posture when doing all this sitting (not to mention all that looking down at your phone or other devices), and, most likely, a workstation that isn't ergonomically designed to help you sit up straight, and you'll suffer as a result—especially with lower back pain. Strong abs will not only help prevent back pain, but they'll boost your stamina, increase your flexibility, *and* make you look and feel amazingly good.

Before you start, there are a few important things to remember:

How your abs will end up looking is predetermined genetically. Don't be discouraged by the Photoshopped images of fantastically flat abs you see in magazines—they're usually doctored images. Some people will quickly get "cut," Magic Mike abs after a short time, and some will do tough abs workouts for years and never attain that kind of definition. What matters is that your abs are strong, and that you take the time to keep them that way.

It's also important that you feel good about your abs. If you are constantly tugging on the shirt by your abs, thinking that's going to help make them look better, it doesn't. It only alerts everyone around you that you aren't confident about your midsection. Be aware of this habit, especially on a job interview or a date. Leave your shirt alone!

Slow and steady is far more effective than rushing through the motions. It's a myth that doing hundreds of fast-paced crunches every day will give you perfect, washboard abs. It's much better to slow down and build up to thirty-second sets of stable, isolated moves that really work.

Here are a few of the best.

## Bike Crunch

DO THIS FOR: At least 3 minutes

SUGGESTED SONG: "Happy" by Pharrell Williams

NOTE: If you have a back injury, be careful and don't do any moves that compromise you.

1. Lie on your back with your hands behind your head and your legs elevated up to a slightly bent 90-degree angle. (How high you can raise them depends on your flexibility—do whatever feels comfortable.)

2. Bring your right elbow toward your left knee, then your left elbow toward your right knee.

3. Keep going till the song is half over.

4. Try to hold the crunch for a two count on each side to force a slower, more concentrated movement until the song ends.

TIPS
- This is going to start to fatigue the muscles in the core, so hold it for as long as you can. If you need to rest, then do so. The more you do this move, the longer you'll be able to hold it.

## Alt Taps

DO THIS FOR: 3 minutes

SUGGESTED SONG: "Blow" by Beyoncé

1. Lie on your back so your body forms an X on the ground.

2. Bring your right hand across to your left foot, then your left hand toward your right foot, lifting your head, neck, and shoulders off the ground.

3. Keep going until the song ends. If you can hit the pace of Beyoncé, great; if you have to half-beat it, fine—but do it!

TIPS
- Yes, it's tough! If you need to rest, then do so.
- If you start to feel it in your neck, it's okay to support it with the hand not in use.
- When you come straight up off the floor, you're working your lower abs. When you twist on an angle, you're working your obliques and your lower abs.

## Ninja Plank Crunch

The plank is one of the only exercises that works the entire core, allowing you to strengthen the front and back of your abdominal area simultaneously. This makes it the most effective exercise in this book, so you should aim for doing it more than any other one!

DO THIS FOR: 3 minutes, 10 seconds
SUGGESTED SONG: "Faith" by George Michael

1. Get into the traditional plank position: forearms on the ground and your body perfectly straight. Lift up so your entire body is off the ground, resting on the weight of your forearms. Do not let your back arch or sag. Stay strong and locked into plank.

2. Bring your right knee forward toward your right elbow, then return to the plank position.

3. Repeat on the left side.

4. Continue for 90 seconds.

5. Rest for 10 seconds.

6. Repeat for 90 seconds more.

TIPS

- Don't look down at your abs; instead, stare in neutral at the floor. Even skinny people look peculiar down there in this position. Don't look—it's weird!

## Grab the Rope

DO THIS FOR: 3 to 4 minutes

SUGGESTED SONG: "The Way You Move" by Big Boi

1. Lie on your back, feet on the ground, knees bent, shoulder width apart.

2. Sit up with your arms and hands reaching through your legs, as if you're grasping for an imaginary rope, and *grab* it as if it's helping you stay up. Your shoulders should be off the ground.

3. Alternate the grab from right to left.

4. Continue for the entire song. Your shoulders and upper back remain up off the floor.

5. When you grab, also turn into the middle, flexing the obliques with each change of the hands. Keep the flex even more into the next move. Stay strong—this shit is hard!

TIPS

- You want a song with a strong, pulsating beat to it, as that will help keep you propelling the grab!

## MY FAVORITE EXERCISES TO REINFORCE HOW YOU LOVE YOURSELF: SG BUTT

What many people don't realize is how connected all our muscles are. All your power starts in your core, then wraps around to the corresponding muscle in the gluteus muscles of your backside (which is the largest muscle group in your body). In other words, you always flex your abs first, brace them, find your balance, and then power through the glutes.

When you go into glute training, you always engage the core first . . . and you really have to think about what move to do next. If you don't, gravity takes over and that's when your lower back starts to hurt. When your mind wanders during any kind of core work, or when you're slouching at your desk, your lower back bears the brunt of this, gets compromised, and starts to ache.

So what does this have to do with love, you might ask? Well, butts are one area of the body where people tend to have a love/hate relationship. I want you to love yours, no matter what shape it's in. Not only because you need strong glutes to keep your body upright and able to move, but because they are so powerful. Loving everything about who you are is one of the most freeing and satisfying things you can accomplish.

## Ballet Barre Squats and Leg Lifts

DO THIS FOR: 5 minutes

SUGGESTED SONG: "Be Alright" by Ariana Grande (x 2)

NOTE: I have been training clients on the barre for thirty years, as it is the most effective and stable place to be. If you don't have access to a barre at a gym, then use a heavy and stable piece of furniture instead.

1. Place your legs a bit farther than hip width apart, toes pointed out.

2. Allow yourself to feel the rhythm of the song while you squat about halfway down to the floor, then come back up to the starting position. Do *not* let your knees go past your toes. If you're super flexible, go deep. If you aren't, stay shallow and build up to going deep!

3. Move over to the barre or piece of furniture and hold on gently with one hand.

4. Turn your foot out as you raise it up. Go to your comfort zone of lifting here—I'm not asking you to punt a football, but almost! Switch legs after you can't bear to do any more. Shoot for 30 on each side.

5. Turn to face the barre or piece of furniture and hold on to it with both hands.

6. Lean forward with your abs tight, then extend one leg out

behind you, toe pointed. Keep your standing leg slightly bent and not locked out. Shoot for 30 on each side.

TIPS

- You most likely started doing moves like this when you were a child. Don't overthink them. Stay connected to your core.
- Imagine your legs long and lean and strong while you are doing the movements.
- Stay positive, and speak nicely to yourself. After just one song of these movements, tomorrow you will feel it!

# Donkey Pee Ballet

DO THIS FOR: 5 minutes

SUGGESTED SONG: Your current favorite song on the radio *or* "New York City" by the Chain Smokers

1. Get down on the floor on all fours.

2. With your heel pointed toward the ceiling, do "donkey kicks" as if you were about to kick someone in the nuts! Make sure to lead with your heel and jam the bottom of that foot up into the air toward the ceiling. Abs tight! Do 30 on each side.

3. Go back to the starting position.

4. Do knee-out-to-the-side raises: Lift your knee up from the hip, abs tight. Squeeze your inner thigh as you move. You

will feel this one so much more in the opposite side booty!
Keep going, 30 each side.

5. Return to the starting position.

6. Do ballet points: Extend one leg back and kick long, straight
back to the wall, abs tight. Push through your second toe
(*not* your big toe). Go for 30 on each side.

TIPS

- This is a classic three-part leg series that really tones
your butt and lengthens your thigh muscles, too. It's an
ideal replacement if you have bum knees and can't do
squats.
- Keep your neck relaxed and in neutral. Take all the
pressure off your back by concentrating on keeping your
abs tight.

# Cardio Fix

DO THIS FOR: 5 minutes

SUGGESTED SONG: Play any fast-paced Madonna here . . . any song with
a strong beat will do.

1. Stand with your feet hip width apart, arms extended in
front you at shoulder height.

2. Crouch down and jump up as high as you can, landing softly.
(This is called a jump squat.) Keep your abs tight. Do 20.

3. Return to the starting position, your arms at your sides, then stand on one leg.

4. Use the force of your arms to jump up in the air, then land softly, balancing on that same leg. Do this 20 times on each side.

5. Return to the starting position, your arms at your sides.

6. Do jumping jacks—except move your legs to the front and back, as if you were cross-country skiing, instead of out to the sides. Try to do this as fast as you can, switching legs, 30 times. (This really turns it up a notch!)

TIPS

* Keep your abs super tight and make sure you breathe calmly. You'll be able to do more this way!

## The Toilet Squat

DO THIS FOR: As long as you like

SUGGESTED SONG: Not appropriate here!

1. Get up from the toilet after you've done your thing and flushed.

2. Do as many squats up and down without touching the toilet seat as you can. Aim for at least 10.

TIPS

- This is one of my favorite exercises, since you're there anyway! Use the moment. You can do it in any bathroom, anywhere, for however long you want to, and it's an effective way to strengthen your glutes and your thigh muscles. It's great on airplanes. Trust me, it's not as easy as it looks.
- Just don't ever touch the toilet with your butt! *Ewww!*

## MY FAVORITE EXERCISES TO GIVE YOU SIGNATURE SG ARMS

When you think about exercise, and moving—going for an energetic walk, perhaps—what comes to mind? Are you just thinking about how a nice, brisk walk will make your cardiovascular system and your leg muscles strong? I hope so. But I also want you to think about the upper half of your body, as arms and shoulders tend to get neglected by those who like to get their aerobic exercise from walking, running, or outdoor cycling. Even if you swim or play racquet sports, you still need to do arm-strengthening exercises regularly—this will make a huge difference in your sporting prowess. And many people get confused about what arm exercises to do, as well as how to do them.

In the cities where I teach, my students are known for their "Stacey Griffith" arms. "My" arms have a special sculpted look, which my students get from the unique directionality of the moves and the sequences I do in class.

I learned decades ago that angles promote angles, so if you want a specific, strong, and sculpted toning to your arms, you not only have to move them in a way that is atypical, but you have to mix up the patterns of movement you make. This will give you the best arms you've ever had—the arms with muscle definition you never thought you'd have—which is especially important for everyone as they grow older and start wondering when that dreaded droop is gonna start, well, drooping!

Before you start, read these important tips:

- How your arms will end up looking is predetermined genetically. (This is true for your abs and butt as well, as you've learned already.) Some people bulk up quickly, and some will always have thinner, leaner muscles.
- It's worth investing in a set of hand weights, especially in one-, two-, and three-pound sizes. Lighter weights—one to five pounds max for women and eight to ten pounds for men—coupled with higher reps are all anyone needs to get the definition they want.
- If you don't have hand weights, you can use full cans of soup or beans, or a large, full bottle of water as a substitute. Anything with some weight to it that fits comfortably in your hands will be fine. Remember this tip next time you're out of town, away from your regular exercise routine or equipment!

- The arms sequence I do in my class usually takes five to seven minutes. This sequence works the biceps, triceps, shoulders, and abs and back. These exercises should be done in the order listed, and should take a couple of minutes each.
- To make yourself even stronger and your arms even better, try to do at least ten push-ups at the end of any arm series. Even if you need to do them from a bent-knee position, a few pushups are better than none. You can also hit planks for two minutes if you want to.
- For the best results and to see your arm muscles really pop, you do have to watch what you eat. This means cutting out the sugar that you get in sodas and desserts, and watching the carbohydrates found in foods like pasta, pizza, and bread! It's not rocket science—it's just discipline. Train your mouth!
- As you do these arm moves, make sure you are thinking about what you want from them and why you are really doing them. This will help you stay on track with your mission.

## Bicep Curl Press

DO THIS FOR: 4 minutes
SUGGESTED SONG: "Sacred Temple" by N.E.R.D.

1. Stand tall, then move your feet shoulder width apart. Hold your weights with your arms down by your sides, palms facing up.

2. With both arms, bring the weights up to a 90-degree angle,

parallel to the floor. As you move, squeeze the sides of your arms as if you are holding a piece of paper on a windy day. Focus more on that squeeze than on actually gripping the weight. (You want to have a relaxed yet sturdy hold on the weight. Be careful not to overgrab.)

3. Next, press the weights over your head as if you are about to put them in the overhead compartment of an airplane. The count is one up, two down (in seconds).

4. Bring your arms back down to the starting position, all the way down to your sides.

TIPS

- Try to do this exercise for the length of one song, but it's okay if you can't at first. If you need to rest, take a short break, then start at the beginning again. Eventually, you'll be able to do all these exercises without stopping.

## Paddle Paddle Paddle

DO THIS FOR: 4 minutes
SUGGESTED SONG: "4 Minutes" by Madonna (ha—perfect song, right?)

1. Keeping your feet shoulder width apart, grip the weights as if you were holding a real paddle for a canoe or a wakeboard and are about to move the paddle through the water on your way back to the shore. Stack one hand on top of the other.

2. Switch the paddle from the right side 8 times to the left side 8 times.

3. Stay in motion, alternating sides, for the duration of the song.

TIPS

- You have to get into this one by slightly bending your legs and really reaching out as if you have the paddle in the water. It will only work if you're really into it.
- If you find that you *can't* get into it, then improvise your own movement like my dad did with his Tai Chi. What's important is that you are reaching out with your upper body, and having some flow with the latissimus, biceps, deltoid, and triceps muscles. This is a full upper-body move, and you should be enjoying it, not dreading it!

# Pour on the Definition

DO THIS FOR: 2 minutes
SUGGESTED SONG: "Pour Some Sugar on Me" by Def Leppard (it fits, right?!)

1. Grab 2-pound weights and sit on the edge of a sturdy chair.

2. Extend the weights straight out, away from your body. Picture a container full of negativity or frustration if you will—whatever it is, use the image as a dump or a get-rid-of moment.

3. Do an imaginary pour as you drop the weights down to your

knees, then turn them upside down as you bring them back up to the starting position.

TIPS

- This is one of my favorite visualization exercises. Picture yourself pouring out whatever you want to get rid of on the way down, then fill up your imaginary container with what you *need* and *want* in your life on the way up. Continue dumping out and filling up for the entire song. The visuals work, but you have to do them. Most people get more caught up in watching themselves in the mirror and focusing on the way they *look*, as opposed to how they could actually make themselves *feel* from the inside out.
- Try doing this with your eyes closed, which I've found can help you focus.

# Floor Flys

DO THIS FOR: 4 minutes
SUGGESTED SONG: "Fly to New York" by Above and Beyond

1. Lie on your back with 2- to 5-pound weights in each hand, arms bent with elbows on the ground, hands up and ready, feet on the floor.

2. Slowly bring your arms straight up in the air until they are up above your forehead.

3. Bring your arms down and wide, almost like you're opening yourself up to receive a big giant hug from down on the

floor. Imagine you're spreading your wings so you can fly as effortlessly as an eagle.

TIPS

- If the 2-pound weights are too heavy at first, try doing this move with no weights at all. Gradually build up to the 1-pound and then the 2-pound weights. You really don't need to go much higher than 2 or 3 pounds once you've mastered it for this exercise to be extremely effective. Guys will want 5 to 10 pounds.
- Keep your abs tight and your back flat on the ground. We tend to lift our butts off the floor, so keep that down, especially the small of your back. Some people also like to place their knees at a 90-degree angle to keep their backs on the floor, so see if that works for you.
- Always have strong, open thoughts when doing this exercise, as you are vulnerable with your heart open and your arms outstretched.

As I quoted Dr. Steinbaum saying earlier in this chapter, mindfulness while exercising is a must. She knows, as I do, that the body follows the mind—so that if your mind is telling your body that it *will* train hard . . . and if you think with every cell in your body about what you're doing . . . and if you stay connected to your movements and your strong breathing patterns . . . and you tell yourself you want to change and you want to be in the best shape of your life and you won't stop until you get there—then you will!

# NINE
## REPEAT

Motivation = Intention + Action

I've written this book because many people may have intent, but can't stick to the action plan that will bring them long-lasting results. I know you are ready to turn that knob—as if it were on an actual door opening toward the changes you've only dreamed of before. Hit the repeat button, and you are unstoppable!

## FIND YOUR SQUAD

I believe that one of the hardest things we can do is show up to our own lives, and show up with energy. We all have times when we aren't motivated and lose interest in living in our Ultimate Center. During these times all you want to do is curl up

"Music is medicine . . . music is vibration . . . music is life."

into a little ball, under the covers, in the dark, and not move. You feel like you just can't do it on your own anymore. You don't know how to propel yourself forward, stick to your plans, or even formulate them properly. You can't believe you're ever going to find motivation again. For whatever reason that may be, we've all been there, and for some people, it actually stops them in their physical tracks.

Let me repeat this: Lack of motivation *stops you in your tracks!* What we need to do is figure out how to get you to move, and that is definitely easier when there are other people around to help you.

That's when you need a squad.

Just as ants can't survive without being in a colony, elephants can't survive without their herd, and dolphins can't survive without their pod, humans can't survive without their squad. We're not solitary creatures. We've evolved and survived to become top of the food chain over thousands of years because we lived in tribes, as squads, and the safety of numbers allowed us to flourish.

I think part of the problem we face in our society is that people feel like they have to tough it out on their own—when in truth the first thing we need to say is, "I need help." Getting help is what friends are for. This is why I loved team sports as a kid, and why I became a group fitness instructor as an adult. I need my squad, I need a team, and I love a group of kick-ass people with high energy. Let's go out and find yours, so you can start kicking some ass, too!

I already showed you that part of empowering yourself to turn your life around is by ridding yourself of toxins—and that includes people. The people who hurt you are not your friends. When I lived in Los Angeles, I felt that a true friend was someone I could call from the airport and tell them I was stranded and they would drop what they were doing and come get me (this doesn't work in New York because so few people have a car). A real friend is a person you can count on, no matter what. They stick by you when you're down. They don't judge you, even when you make really dumb mistakes. A true friend like that is the heart of your squad.

I think people put up with so much shit from other people because they're so afraid of *not* having someone love them that they allow toxicity to stay. Why would you want to have members of your squad who are always putting you down, are unreliable, or untrustworthy? How can you move forward and have confidence that you can attain your goals and stay motivated when someone is dragging you down?

Like attracts like—your squad should be like-minded people. Not just your personalities or the kind of jobs you have—because I know people who are very different yet as close as identical twins who just *get* each other.

Another great quality to look for in your squad are people who will tell you the truth, and not "yes" you just for the sake of avoiding confrontation. I learned in my relationship that arguing and disagreeing are okay, and part of personal growth is debating with someone. I learned a lot about

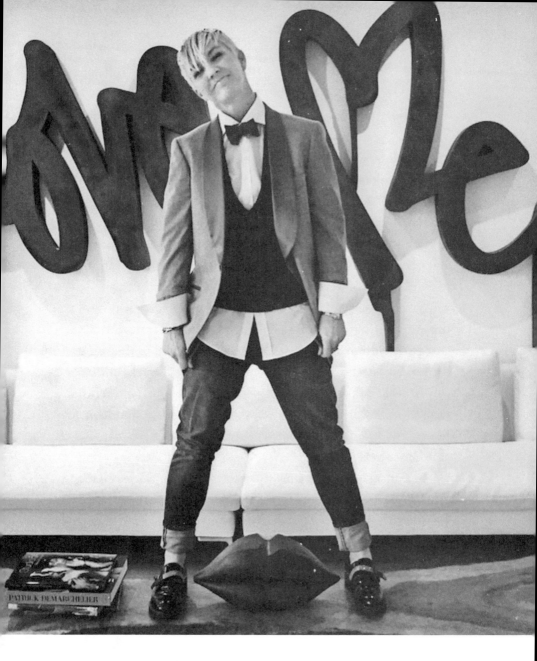

Bruno Cucinelli

myself by sitting in some uncomfortable truths with my partner, and because we were honest with each other, we actually got *closer* through a lot of arguments. Learning to sit in
them doesn't mean anyone is leaving—it just means they care
enough to be honest.

That's why finding your squad and becoming an active par-
ticipant in it is often the difference between staying motivated
and giving up. Human beings are social creatures, after all.
It's why houses of worship are there for those who need to pray;
why groups like AA help addicts fight their demons; why having a dinner party for your friends is so much fun; why sitting in a stadium and screaming encouragement to the home
team is so satisfying; and why my classes are always full. It's
why fitness or dance classes are, for many, so much more fun
than solitary workouts. We feed off one another's common interests. We understand what brought us together. We fuel one
another's energy needs.

The concept of finding my squad has been ingrained in me
since I was eight, when I started playing team sports. I joined
the soccer team because that's where my friends were. Yes, I
quickly got good at the game, but what really mattered to me
was being with the people I cared about. That's what kept me
going on days when I was tired or stressed or just didn't feel
like playing. I didn't want to let my team down.

Finding your own squad will provide energy to keep you going . . . and going . . . and going. Whether your squad is in your
fitness studio or at a support group or in your book club or at a

"SG = squad goals"

When you feel stuck and in need of some motivation, creating a new accountability squad—or fine-tuning your current squad—can give you the energy, courage, and companionship you need. Here's how to start forming your new squad—the one that will help you keep your resolve:

- Go through all the players in your life and pick the starting five. These are the ones you trust the most; the ones who share your goals and dreams. They will get you motivated to work out and go to the gym with you. They will show you how to cook a healthy dinner in less than twenty minutes and invite you to places you've never been before.
- Pick a goal to achieve with your squad. It could be twenty workout classes in twenty days, or white-water rafting in June, or climbing Mount Kilimanjaro on New Year's Eve. Or just walking together every day in your neighborhood, rain or shine.
- Begin training for that goal, with your squad, and hold one another accountable for the end results.

FORMING A NEW
ACCOUNTABILITY SQUAD

coffeehouse—or even just hanging out with you on a lazy day. A squad is there to get you up and out the door. They are the moral support and encouragement you need.

I have been so blessed throughout my life and career to find amazing squads. We have gone on long-distance bike rides for days on end, through two countries, and through three states. We've lived in India and traveled all over the world. I've seen thousands of students a year for the last decade. I'm *lucky*. You

As energetic as I am normally, some days are just a drag, and they drag me down. Maybe I'm getting a cold, or have jet lag, or I just didn't get my much-needed seven hours of sleep the night before. Am I going to let my students know how I feel? No way. I'm in that room to give them everything I've got, and they expect that from me. I'm gonna kick the ass off the blahs.

So when I'm having one of those days, I might take a slightly longer nap than usual. Or I'll add a packet of e-boost powder to my bottle of water, and that can make me really feel better quickly. A few blueberries also seem to give me a little boost.

And I know that by the end of the day, my energy will have returned. Why? Because the rooms I teach in are supercharged. You walk in, and you will literally feel the adrenaline of all my students zinging off the walls. The energy is flowing; it hits you in the face with the nicest kind of smack of positivity. But it's something more. It's the *intention* that floods the room. Everyone comes to class prepared to work it, and to work it hard. The resonance of all that intention lingers. It feels *amazing*. It helps everyone work with even more purpose than they thought possible.

You can feel how rooms are supercharged in all sorts of locations, of course. In a cathedral or a small chapel; in a library reading room or a museum; in a theater when the lights dim and the curtain goes up. It's all about how a specific environment elicits collective intentions. And this is why a lot of people prefer to work out by taking classes or going to a gym. Any space devoted to movement is going to be supercharged, and will automatically make you feel more energized, too.

So how do you find somewhere to energize yourself off the collective vibe? Especially if you're more into solitary workouts? I had to really think about an answer, because I've always been on sports teams and I've always preferred to be part of a group workout. You know that old saying, "Once you get there, you'll be fine"? I always tell my students that getting to class is the hardest part. Obviously it's my job, and I have to be there, I add, so they should be a lot more excited than I am, because I'm at work and they're not!

My suggestion is that you ask a friend or friends who go to classes or group workouts if you could join them. Be sure to introduce yourself to the instructor and say that you've never done this kind of group exercise before and you're a little nervous. A good teacher will be kind and reassuring as well as encouraging. Take a few deep breaths. Set your intentions. Keep your mind open. One of your intentions should be to just relax during this time that you are devoting to yourself, to enjoy it even if you need a little guidance or correction while you're learning new moves.

Then do the workout and see how you feel. I bet you are going to surprise yourself—because the energy of the group is going to fuel your own workout in a way that's just not possible when you do it on your own. It might not be as satisfying to you as your long, solo runs or bike rides, but it certainly is a different kind of vibe that I hope you'll realize can complement your regular workouts. The only way to experience this is to actually get out there and do it!

HOW THE ENERGY OF THE GROUP CAN ENERGIZE YOU

know that already. And now I want you to feel lucky, too. You are a human being, not an inanimate object—that, to me, is so incredibly lucky!

## YOU CAN'T MAKE A PUPPY A DOG

When I was in my early twenties, a lot of my friends were becoming very successful. They owned homes and nice cars. They traveled a lot and had disposable income. I wanted to be like them, but I just wasn't. I was a high school dropout, so I didn't have many options other than the manual-labor jobs you get when you're a dropout. I painted houses, I was a personal trainer, I worked in retail, and I was a cocktail waitress. I worked hard. And then, when I was twenty-six years old, I got a job as a salesperson at my local Family Fitness Center, which was part of a chain. I loved my job so much. It was a really good fit for me at the time.

Whenever there was a company meeting, they would talk about peaking. This is how they explained it: When you fill the pipeline full of clients and referrals that are passing your name along, that will help grow the business and your cash flow. But, they told us, you can't make a puppy a dog. You have to *grow* into being a dog. You can't just become a dog. You have to grow. The years have to go by until you become a dog—and that's the *peak*.

When they talked about filling the pipeline and pushing, I would get so frustrated because I knew I had it in me, but I also knew that I was still the puppy and there was nothing I could do to make myself grow faster into being the dog. I tried to speed up the process anyway. Oh, did I hustle. I'd get to that gym at five thirty in the morning and I'd go up to all the people already working out on the treadmills, and I'd give them a guest pass and tell them to bring their friends.

The gym was smart and awarded a prize every month for the top salesperson. In June, the top salesperson would win a mountain bike. And I really wanted the mountain bike because I couldn't afford to buy my own. I'd be rolling calls for hours, telling clients or newbies that they won a free guest pass to the gym. The next month, the prize was a weekend in Catalina, and I really wanted to go to Catalina but I couldn't afford it, so I would roll calls for hours on end and sign up new members. The next month, the prize was a day at the spa. It was the perfect prize because I'd get two massages in one day.

My strategies worked, but when I kept winning, my colleagues got mad. They thought it wasn't fair that I won the prizes every month, and decided the award-giving was rigged. They said I was stealing leads or going around and taking the names out of the membership boxes. I was steamed. "You know what?" I told them. "I invested in my own membership boxes and I put them in all of the local businesses and I established a relationship with those people and I filled the pipeline. I did the work."

What I didn't say—but what I knew in my heart—was that this couldn't possibly be my peak, even though I was a champion salesperson. I knew for sure it wasn't my peak when someone told me that at other gyms, salespeople were making $10,000 a month. I could not believe somebody actually made that kind of commission selling gym memberships. Then my friend Marcus told me that the aerobics teacher was making even more money. I remember thinking, *Wow, I don't know if I could do that. That aerobic teacher's really got it together.* She was super organized. Every song was perfectly placed.

At the time, to me that was the epitome of ultimate control. And now that's exactly what I do when I teach. I'm not the puppy anymore. The puppies might know what the pieces are, but they don't yet have the wisdom and experience to put them all together. It took me many years, but I know that I've finally grown into the dog I was meant to be.

What I learned was that if you feel like you're about to peak or have peaked, you need to find another peak. (Look at Warren Buffett. He didn't make his first million until he was fifty-three, and he's now one of the richest men in the world.) I would climb one peak, find a new, higher peak, and then, when I was ready, start climbing again.

In other words, your intentions, goals, and life are not about one solitary peak. Your life is a whole range of mountains. You're going to go up and down. For almost everything in life, for every positive there is a negative, for every push there's a pull. (Everything is in twos—which is why this book is called *Two Turns from Zero*.) Dealing with this duality is what you should try to focus on, because if what you're doing isn't working one way, it's going to work a different way. If you're down from one peak you know you were up before, look at the next peak and ask yourself how you're going to go up again. Get your MAP and figure out the route. It's a different journey to another peak.

*As long as you keep moving.*

## MOVEMENT = MOTIVATION

Movement is what's going to make the changes in your life start showing up. *Moving* is what sets the energy in everything in motion. It's not just you moving the ideas in your head around or moving from one house to another—it's getting your *body* in motion, which is the most important trigger for you to LET the sunshine in. To Love, Eat, Train, Repeat. Over and over, in perpetual motion, until you find the Ultimate Center.

In other words, your thoughts, goals, and dreams have to be backed up with action. Not just the everyday action that gets you out of the house. The kind of action that pushes you out of your comfort zone. Let's take this book as an example. I am a high school dropout, as you know. It was a struggle for me to go back to the classroom as a twenty-year-old to finish high school, but I did it. It was uncomfortable and embarrassing. Thank God I did, and my beloved grandma Stella still has that diploma up on her wall to remind me of that accomplishment. The thought of writing an entire book was something that seemed out of my realm of possibility. So I got help.

My coauthor, Karen, and I talked and wrote and had endless

back-and-forths for months, in person, on the phone, and on the computer. The more we worked, and as the book took shape, the more I realized that not only was I enjoying it, I was doing more writing and editing than I ever thought I could do—and I was good at it! Me, the worst student in the world! I mean, if you'd asked any of my teachers if they ever thought I could do this, they would have said, "Yes, Stacey . . . if you *apply* yourself." That was my demise in school—application and effort. For school I had zip; for sports I had 110 percent. First kid to practice, last kid out of the gym. I would sweep and mop the basketball court when I got there. I would put all the balls away when I left. I was the coaches' pet on every team, and MVP on most. I *wanted* it, and I always did what it took to get it. I found my skill set, and I focused on it. The problem was that I didn't like learning anything from a book. How ironic that I am writing one.

The best conversation Karen and I had when we started working together took place in a car. I had to go downtown to a photo shoot, so we got in the car the studio had sent, and we headed down New York's FDR Drive, along the East River. *We* weren't actually moving, but we were *in motion* (there aren't any stoplights on the FDR, so we didn't get stuck in traffic). It was one of those incredible experiences where, literally, two people who didn't know each other all that well yet just looked at each other and *bam!* Out flew the ideas. I was able to articulate exactly what I wanted this book to be.

The entire ride couldn't have been more than twenty-five minutes or so, but they were twenty-five indelible minutes.

After that, I had the confidence to move forward. Whenever I felt stuck, I just visualized the feeling of that car ride, the ideas zooming out of my head, and the wonderful, deep satisfaction that what I wanted to share with the world could, in fact, be shared outside of my classes. It was just incredible.

Movement always enhances learning. I said this earlier in the book—good professors or lecturers are always in motion; they're pacing back and forth as they talk. That's because if you look at the actual structure of the brain, the motor cortex is located in the Broca area, attached to the section of the brain that handles speech. When you make any kind of movement, it goes back and forth to the Broca area. It's all connected.

The best professionals in any realm know this. Actors and musicians rehearse. Speakers and teachers go over their notes. Models walk up and down the catwalk before a fashion show. Athletes, in particular, know this. At some Olympic events, for example, you'll see the athletes, especially divers and gymnasts, literally walking themselves through their routines, in place, before they do them. Why? *They were physically embodying their creative visualizations.* My inspiration, Tony Robbins, was famous for doing this with tennis player Andre Agassi. He made Andre go through the entire match of the US Open point by point until he won. From the very first point to every volley and every single point. Game, set, match.

These athletes moved like this not to make themselves feel invincible, but because they knew they needed the utmost preparation. They had a plan. MAP it out. Make a Plan. Visualize what you want. State your intentions. But don't think that just stating things will bring you everything you want. Yes, it is the ideal start. But it's still up to you to give yourself that burst of energy and get you moving to make your words real. Get going. Make moves toward the MAP by calling, texting, e-mailing, carrier pigeon—whatever it takes. Talk and talk and write it down and follow through!

MAP-ing it out allows you to expect the unexpected. You've thought things through. You know what can go right and/or wrong. Your preparation gives you flexibility. You're in a state of what I like to call Flex Appeal.

When I went to India to study yoga, I was *so* not flex. But after two months, I could wrap my arms around the bottom of my feet, and do a handstand, a back bend, and all kinds of other crazy shit I never thought I could do. All I did was stretch every day, because that's why I was there; I had an intention to get good at it, so the motivation was behind it. That gave me Flex Appeal—physically and emotionally.

One of my students, "Matty Moo," told me a dramatic story of how flexibility saved his life. He'd been a regular in my class for years, and was also an avid yogi and experienced skier. When he had a traumatic fall on the slopes—he hit a lift pole between his neck and his shoulder; I know, *ow!*—the ski patrol arrived with the stretcher, expecting to find a body, and couldn't believe he was still breathing. Not only was he still alive, but the doctors at the hospital told him he'd survived and would have a much speedier recovery because he was in such superior physical condition. They could tell even after an accident that he was lithe and strong. Flex Appeal saved his life.

Flexible people are more successful than tightly wound ones. Tightly wound people use vocabulary like "I can't," "I won't," or "That hurts." Flexible people change their language and their muscles. They start to say things like, "I can," "I will," and "This feels good." Flex Appeal is a metaphor for how we have to live our lives and inhabit our bodies. To be flexible is to be ready to change and take on new challenges and grow. It means being ready to twist and turn and not get hurt.

I want you to find new solutions and keep learning, because that, too, will increase your Flex Appeal.

## Visualization for Motivation

This is an excellent visualization for forward-thinking and to make you feel safe.

1. Sit comfortably and close your eyes. Imagine that your body is a house or an apartment that you're renovating. You weren't able to actually go see the renovations take place because you had too many other commitments. Picture yourself in winter, with cold and snow, and then spring, with rain showers and flowers poking themselves out of the ground, and today is the day you're finally going to see your new and improved home. The home of your dreams.

2. Take your time walking up to this new home. Savor the anticipation. Be as thrilled and excited as a little child opening up the birthday presents and blowing out the candles.

3. Turn the knob and open the door. There it is. The new and improved home you've wanted all your life. Everything you've dreamed of is there.

4. Celebrate your renovation. Bask in how amazing that feels. Run your fingers over the shiny woodwork and the smooth texture of the paint on your walls. Smile at how perfectly these renovations match your vision.

5. Drop your chin, and as you do, feel the gentle stretch open up the back of your neck. See your best self, standing there in the sexy, strong, and confident body you know you belong in.

Take as much time as you can give here in this meditation. Think about what is going to happen after you open your eyes. Go through the checklist of motivation tools that you've already learned in the book. Take this time right now to reinvigorate your spirit, turn all systems on inside, and when you open your eyes, you will have the power and energy to go out there and take care of the things you need to take care of. Do it *now!*

I have always been a dreamer, a fantasizer, a wanderer of thoughts. It's something I can't control; it's part of what makes me the creative channel I am. Some of my thoughts make absolutely no sense, and some are pure delicious creativity. I encourage you to try to channel and practice your creative thoughts, keeping in mind the difference between reality, fantasy, and goal-oriented visions. The more realistic you are in your thought process during your meditations, the better chance the universe has for lining them up "with" you. In my belief, if they're going to get caught by the universe, they're going to have to match 100 percent of your reality.

Thinking about motivation reminds me of a story my friend Gina told me about her college days, when she decided to do something she'd always wanted—to get stronger and row on the crew team. "At the first meeting, we sat in the dusty old gym, and the coach was describing the kind of workouts we'd have, where the boats were, and the commitment we'd need to make," she said. "One of my classmates was sitting off to the side, listening intently. She was overweight, but she had this look on her face that I can still picture clearly, decades later. It was the face of pure determination. It was almost as if I could read her thoughts, because I could tell just by looking at her that she was going to go far. She was *fierce*. Something in her had clicked. She didn't want to be in that body anymore. By the end of the year, she'd dropped fifty pounds. She was buffer than buff. Even better, she'd become the captain of the crew team. I was so proud of her—and she was a lot prouder of herself. She'd earned that right!"

I often see this look of pure determination on the faces of my students. One of my favorite things as a teacher is to see

**By Super Body Super Brain author Michael Gonzalez-Wallace**

I'd heard about the energy, music, enthusiasm and motivation in Soul-Cycle classes many times over the years. When I finally decided to go, I was lucky that I had a unique instructor, Stacey Griffith.

As a professional in the fitness field for more than twenty years, I knew the drill. I was not expecting to encounter such an inspirational instructor, however—one who not only connected mind, body, and soul, but who was also able to connect the three in more of a metaphysical form where past, present, and future coexist simultaneously (as our old, much-admired professor Albert Einstein would express in his theory of relativity). Yes, these concepts can be applied to exercise as well, but it is a very rare fitness instructor who is able to bring them together.

Stacey's music selection and her complete emotional involvement while she's teaching go beyond that of a regular instructor. Every beat, every exercise had a point where it was a clear "Come on," and you had to do it and do it well. There was no way you would decide not to do it.

At some point in the class, Stacey talked, almost in a holistic way, about how we are all part of a continuum . . . an ongoing process where love, health, work, and friendship are in perpetual motion. Constantly moving. If we refuse to accept this irrefutable law of life, then this is what will make us get stuck. If, on the other hand, we are able to adjust dynamically and engage in the continuum process of perpetual motion, then this is where we are able to transform our lives from the inside out. Deciding to take class and work hard that day—or deciding to engage in any form of exercise on any given day—was exactly part of that dynamic process.

What surprised me the most was that Stacey's energy level was extremely high and her words strong, yet she always remained calm. She reminded me of the best basketball coaches I'd had when I played semiprofessionally in Spain. No matter how tense the game was, the good coaches remained calm and in control. They knew they needed to do so in order to make clear decisions with a focused mind and a serene heart.

I also realized something during class. I was getting chills from the combination of cycling in such a darkened room, coupled with the sensory activation of that inner sixth sense, those messages from the divine, that we all have—but that are often interfered with or ignored when there is, literally, too much light. Stacey's class took me right back to the past, to the year 2000, back in Madrid, Spain. At that time I was an investment banker, working at Santander Bank. The gym I used to attend in Madrid was called Holiday Inn. One day—actually it was Saturday, September 8, which I remember with perfect clarity so many years later—I showed up for my usual Spinning class at eight A.M. It was one of my favorite classes, as it wasn't just riding the bike but incorporated push-ups and entire body movements like Stacey's class does.

The room was packed, and the clock was ticking. The instructor didn't show, and people were starting to get frustrated. I asked Diana, the manager, if I could take over, and she said sure. I was so happy afterward, and luckily my fellow riders were, too, and I was then asked to teach three Spinning classes every week. I was a banker by day, Spinning instructor by night! I moved to New York City a few years later, and I always wonder what would have happened had I not gotten up to teach the class that night. I don't know if I would have shifted from a successful career in finance to an even more successful career in fitness. Spinning is what did it for me. *(cont.)*

HOW STACEY GETS ME MOTIVATED

**HOW STACEY GETS ME MOTIVATED**

I was so grateful that Stacey brought back those memories into a workout where past, present, and future became intertwined and brought out the best in me.

At the end of Stacey's class, I was in the zone. I was performing at that challenging level that for me, as a former athlete, I want and need to be challenged to reach. My heart rate monitor showed that I'd burned 568 calories with my heart rate averaging 140. That was great—but it was the emotional and psychological benefits that my state-of-the-art wearable technology, blinking on my wrist, was not able to quantify.

In other words, it was the combination of motivation, psychology, and movement that coalesced into the perfect mojo for me. Stacey's "Come on!" was just the snap I needed to move from a static to a dynamic performance.

And here's the best thing about what I learned in class that day. You don't have to be Spinning in the room with Stacey to benefit from the power and the motivation she gives her students. You just have to read this book!

someone who is out of shape but has the steely-eyed look as they start riding—the muscles might not be toned yet, but the attitude is there. That is a person who is going to succeed. And I would much rather teach students like that than the most physically fit students who have the attitude that they're stuck on the bike. They're just phoning it in. When I see that, I want to say, "Coming here to this class was your choice. It was a premeditated choice because you had to reserve the bike a week ago. You set this up. So come on! What are you waiting for?"

## THE *TOYA*, AKA THE EASIEST, MOST EMPOWERING EXERCISE YOU CAN DO ANYWHERE

The Spanish word for "towel" is *toalla*, but I've adapted the phonetic spelling of "toya" to name this exercise, which I'm putting here, in the final chapter, as something that will make you stronger, anytime, anyplace, using an object found in your home or hotel room, or that can easily be stashed in a desk drawer or in your car. If you only do one song before you leave the house for the day, or when you want a burst of energy, engaging your body and getting moving will help set your intentions and bring better clarity to your thoughts. It takes so little to give you so much!

### Stacey's *Toya* Arms

DO THIS FOR: 4 ½ to 5 minutes
SUGGESTED SONG: "Uptown Funk" by Bruno Mars

1. Hold a hand towel lengthwise by the corners and bunch it up in 2-inch increments so that it looks like a bar. Stand with your feet shoulder width apart, knees comfortably bent.
2. With your elbows bent at a 90-degree angle, turn your palms facing out. Keep your shoulders back, chin up, and abs tight. To the beat, pretend you're facing a clock, then

move your arms side to side as if you are hitting the 3 and the 9 on the clock. Your elbows should be steady. Do this for 1 minute.

3. Move your right hand up to the imaginary 12 o'clock position, and swirl the towel around with your left hand as if you're beating eggs. Do this for 1 minute, then switch hands and swirl to the other side.

4. Move your arms straight arms up over, then bend your elbows at a 90-degree angle so your hands and the towel are behind your head. Press up with straight arms and then back again (like a shoulder press) for 30 seconds. Your hands stay behind your head.

5. Bring the towel in front and wrap it around one hand like a big bandage, then hit out at a pretend punching bag at shoulder height for 1 minute. Wrap the towel around the other hand and repeat for 1 minute.

TIPS

- When I get to step 5, I am really going for the punches. I used to imagine I was punching the cancer cells out of my dad so he'd heal.

- You can also do this to a slower beat as a sort of Moving Meditation. If, for example, I need ideas for a project or have writer's block, or need to break a cycle and I know something has to give, I like to ask the universe to get something started. Step 3 is particularly useful for creating an imaginary whirlpool of energy that is instantly energizing.

What *are* you waiting for?

When you finish this book and put it down on your table, the next step is totally up to you. The next step and the next level are out there waiting for you. I know you're ready to reach out and grab it. Leave this book where it's easy to see, so you can pick it up at any time, and thumb through until you stop on a page. Think of it as your motivational Tarot card reading. Whatever page you land on was the page you were meant to read that day!

Did you ever see the movie *Kill Bill 2*? Near the end, Uma Thurman's character finds the über-assassin Bill, played by David Carradine, and when he tries to kill her, she gets to him first, leaving him fatally wounded. Knowing he's about to meet his fate, he stands up and asks her how he looks. What does she say in response? "You look *ready.*"

Being ready means you'll be able to drive around any roadblocks on your way forward, because you know that nothing is going to stop you from getting to your destination. I always think to myself when I'm leaving the house that if I feel good on the inside, there's no need to double-check myself in the mirror. I'm just gonna go with it! I think if you're feeling awesome, go with awesome. Check yourself in the mirror in the morning so you look the way you want, obviously. I do this, set my intentions, and hit the road.

I hope this book will plant seeds for your future—that I've sparked your interest and fired the connections in your very capable brain. I hope I've shown you how to make different choices, and to use the power you already have in your head to do creative visualizations and Moving Meditations.

The ultimate happiness will come to you, because you have the ultimate control. Over your feelings, your moods, your dreams, your work. Many of my students ask me how I got to the place where I am now, and how I'm able to teach with seemingly 100 percent in every class. "I've never had a bad class with you," they tell me, "and you're never in a bad mood." That always makes me laugh, because I *am* in a bad mood sometimes—but not in my office and not in my classes. Because I don't bring my issues into the room. That is real control! I set my intentions for the day, and I find the determination to bring them to reality.

With the right motivation in your life, you're gonna nail every audition or job interview or meeting with your kids' teachers in school. You can't be off your game in those meetings. Leave your cell phone in your bag. You can't be tapping your foot or chewing your fingernails or exuding anxiety or worry. You have to be chill in those meetings. Sometimes you will get frustrated or furious, but you need to just put on a heartfelt smile and say, "Chill, I'm cool," and then face it. So whatever you have to deal with, right now, or in an hour, or for the rest of today, I want you to say to yourself, "Chill, I'm cool."

Your new way of thinking is your wealth. It's not about the things you have—it's about how you feel in your body, how amazing you feel every single day of your life. I know you're

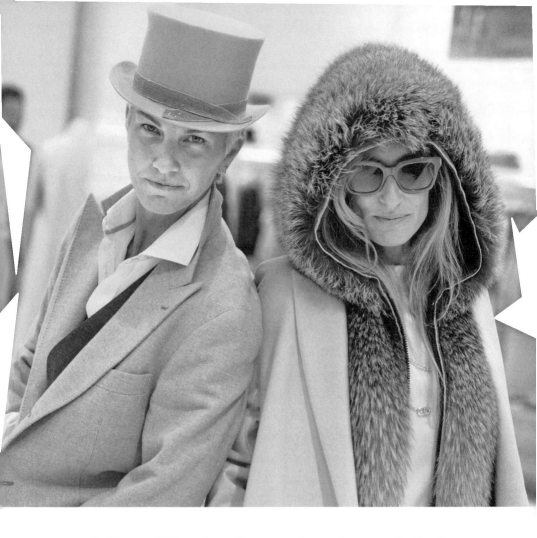

ready. You could have been born a rock or a tree, or a body of water or a fish swimming in it. But you are a human being and have the ability to change people's lives. To make people feel comfortable and loved and wanted. To make yourself feel that way, too. You were born ready or you never would have made it into this universe, with endless possibilities for success.

Don't stop thinking about what you want. What you want to

achieve is in your capable hands. Think about what you want, and send it up, out there to the universe. That's where we send everything we want: *Up.*

I am so proud of you for pushing through it. It's not easy. *Why?* Because *easy doesn't change you.* Think about all those difficult decisions you've had to make in your life, and how stronger you became after they were done. After you got through them you looked back in amazement that you ever found your way through. But you did. I *never* thought I would be able to live a sober life. Now I don't know how I ever *didn't!*

Determination gets you through it, focus gets you through it, drive gets you through it, tenacity gets you through it, will gets you through it, desire gets you through it, love gets you through it, light definitely gets you through it!

Close your eyes and feel a moment alone with yourself, feel the stronger version of you that you worked so hard to maintain, fuel, and energize. Take this moment right now, and come back in ten seconds.

Sprint into your life toward your goals and dreams. When you start feeling creative feelings, when you start thinking of amazing ideas, you have to put them in motion. Your creative process is your success in your life.

I was at an amusement park a while ago with a group of friends, and there's nothing I love more than going on the highest, wackiest, most scream-inducing roller coaster. One of my friends turned green just at the sight of the tracks, and he said he'd sit it out. He went to get a drink, and by the time

I found him I'd ridden the coaster. Three times. "You're done already?" he asked. "Yep," I replied. "And I'm gonna go ride it *again*." It's the thrill of the ride.

Turning yourself two turns from zero and toward your Ultimate Center has nothing to do with anybody else but you. This is *your* life. Look how strong you are when you put your mind to it. Look how strong you are when you set your goals and hit them. You know how amazing that feels. When you're ready, just turn the knob and go into the life that you know you were meant to be living.

You're in it to win it. You have your squad. You have your intentions set. You have your MAP. Determination always takes you to the end. Be determined in your efforts with *everything* in your life.

I'll leave you with this: If I can come from the depths of addiction, broke as a bum, cars repossessed, traffic warrant arrests, bills, zero zero *zero* effort to improve myself, and end up as one of the top fitness professionals in the world, you can also accomplish whatever it is you want for yourself.

I found my squad in fitness. I rose up into honesty and stopped using things that hurt me, and fueled myself with things that fired me up. I found my passion in teaching, and I know that you'll find your passion in what your interests are, too, and then go for it. *Can't stop won't stop pushing. Can't stop won't stop changing.* Here we go. . . .Join my SGuad at twoturns fromzero.com/.

TWO TURNS FROM ZERO STARTS NOW.

# ACKNOWLEDGMENTS

Deb, without you, Jenna, Cloe, and Lilli, I could never have had a foundation strong enough to write this book.

I want to thank my mom and dad for making me. Dad, I know we talked about this the last week you were on this earth, and it's finally here—so enjoy it in heaven with my little brother, Seanny. Mom, you really taught me compassion and love, and that has been at the center of my teaching since I began. Thank you.

Tiff, Julye, Griff, and Emz, I love you so much. Sandy Lynch, for taking care of my grandma with such love. Thanks for being my family. You have no choice!

Grandma Stella, for teaching me that working hard and staying in shape are important. Trying things without "askin' what's in 'em" is fine. Take risks, get rest, and wash your face. Then finish what you started. Finally . . . I finished something great!

Elizabeth and Julie, thank you for believing we could create magic together, even when the music was too loud on Seventy-Second Street. Thank you for trusting what I was up to on the other side of the frosted glass door.

E, you're the best wing wifey around. Without you I'm a mess!

Thanks to my entire incredible team: Winston, Lauren, Margaret, Benjamin, and Suzanne.

To my publishing squad of Henry Ferris and Kathy Gordon, thank you for your loyalty and faith that we could create something life-changing!

I want to thank Geralyn Lucas and Lily Neumeyer for the countless hours they spent helping me kick-start this book.

Thank you to Meredith Geller, Dr. Suzanne Steinbaum, and Michael Gonzalez-Wallace for their brilliant contributions to this book.

Thank you to ALL my SoulCycle family. You know who you are without my saying!

To all of my LA friends who have witnessed the "cracker" become a responsible adult.

And to every single one of my students over the last two decades, I hope we can continue on this journey together to the end of fitness time. Some of you started as students, became friends, and have become chosen family.

Eighty-Third Street is my home. The Hamptons is my peace. Thank you.

Happiness, joy, love, and light, Deepak . . . you are a divine being.

Oh, and thank you, Oprah, for being my beacon of awesome. And Kelly Ripa for your loyalty and effervescence every year for a decade.